Dear Bruno,

With my best wishes for a
life filled with abundant
WHealth!

Roddy

BodyWHealth

JOURNEY TO ABUNDANCE

BodyWHealth

JOURNEY TO ABUNDANCE

Roddy Carter, MD

Aquila Life Science Press
La Jolla, California

FIRST AQUILA LIFE SCIENCE PRESS EDITION, DECEMBER 2015
Published by Aquila Life Science, LLC, La Jolla, CA

BODYWHEALTH.

ISBN: 978-0-9969889-0-2

Printed in the United States of America

To Karen, Matthew, Michael, Kirstin, and Robyn,

I love you more than life itself.

CONTENTS

ACKNOWLEDGEMENTS

I did not invent BodyWHealth. I didn't even discover it. I was merely given the keys to unlock it. My greatest thanks go to the unseen powers that have gifted each of us with the birthright of abundance, have given me knowledge of the keys that unlock it, and have inspired me with courage to share this insight with you. Doing so will be my lasting honor.

I have met many wonderful, interesting travelers on my journey. I have learned something from each interaction. My life is a rich tapestry of insights and knowledge from these engagements. I am extraordinarily grateful for the encouragement and support of my many patients, clients, colleagues, and friends. To each of you, thank you.

Two special colleagues have worked closely with me to create this book.

Sarah Dawson is a talented editor. She has balanced curiosity with discipline. She has been a coach and a cheerleader. She has treated my bad ideas gently, and my good ideas with respect. She has helped me to articulate the pathway to Abundance. Sarah, thank you for your delicate, firm literary leadership.

Jolie Kalfaian is an insightful book designer. She has brought aesthetics to the BodyWHealth story and helped us to translate the concept into a clean, warm visual experience. She has helped me to illustrate the pathway to Abundance. Jolie, thank you for your empathetic, focused creative leadership.

My most intense gratitude is reserved for my wonderful wife, Karen, and my beautiful children, Matthew, Michael, Kirstin, and Robyn. You have been inspiring, generous, and patient. You encouraged my personal journey to BodyWHealth, and you enabled my writing of this book, helping me to put guidance and knowledge into the hands of our fellow travelers on this beautiful road.

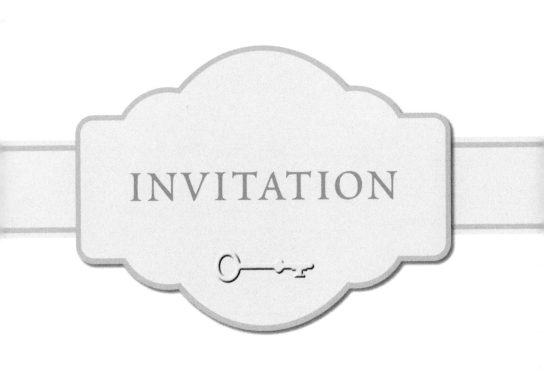

INVITATION

Five years ago, I was five years older. No, that's not a mistake. Five years ago, I was five years *older*! I actually gained a year of youth for each of the past five years. Today, I am ten years younger than I was destined to be.

Despite being a very-well-trained physician, knowledgeable about living a healthy life, I was living in the dark back then. I was a train wreck waiting to happen. I was grossly overweight, couldn't drag myself up two flights of stairs without gasping, and slept poorly. I couldn't enjoy my body and had no pride in its appearance. More than all of that, I was unhappy! I hauled myself through each day, trying to salvage what was left of my dying embers. As I aged, I thought, *I must work harder. I must get a better job, a better salary, a better bonus, and build my wealth.* I thought that, in the absence of vitality, at least more money would give my life meaning.

I couldn't have been more wrong. One day, I stepped off a grueling transcontinental flight. I had spent the past several hours feeling choked to death in my seat. The discomfort of the restrictive seat belt exaggerated the internal agony I already had over my degenerating state. It was a moment of desperation; I knew I couldn't go on the same way. I decided—not for the first time, for sure—that I had to make a change.

But this time was different from any previous attempts to grab the reigns of my escaping youth. For me, it was where I started my journey to WHealth, a destination more valuable than health or wealth alone. This time, unlike any time before, I went back to my scientific roots. I drew on my deep biological insight, basing my recovery on the very science that was working against me in that moment. I understood deeply and profoundly within myself that I had a biological imbalance; the fires of degeneration and decay were raging, and I had to stop them. With the science of habit on my side, I started the journey to reboot my life into something good.

I won't lie. The beginning was hard…until an immensely powerful discovery changed everything. Standing alone scrutinizing myself in my bedroom mirror, I suddenly saw an athlete. An out-of-shape athlete, perhaps, but an athlete nonetheless. And that athlete deserved to be treated as such, both physically and emotionally. By complete accident, I had discovered a power that we all have dormant within us, suppressed though it might be: the power of belief. From that moment forward, I *believed* I was an athlete and behaved that way, even though it still took my body time to catch up. Being a scientist, I went back to the emerging body of scientific knowledge to understand this ubiquitous but grossly underused power of belief. It might be the most valuable thing I will share with you over the course of our journey together.

When I unlocked this power, my own journey leaped forward. With joy and excitement, and very tangible results, I galloped toward WHealth with my brain leading the charge. Within a few months, I had tasted it, and there was no going back.

To my immense surprise, on my journey to health, I also found happiness. The physician and scientist in me had sought physical health. In that process, as a reward for my diligence and perseverance, I unlocked intimate links between body and mind and emotion. By honoring the foundational chemistry of physical health, I unlocked emotional health. I discovered that Mother Nature intends this in her primal design for us.

Today, I celebrate my youthful body. I know that I can and will stay young. I know that decay is a choice, and I have chosen against it. I know that my greatest investment is in life itself. I am still on the BodyWHealth journey. The wonderful thing about this journey is that it's not over once you taste victory. In many ways, that's only the beginning. I know that health and happiness are the building blocks of prosperity, a state of profound fulfillment wherein we are recognized and rewarded for the value we bring to the world. Prosperity knows no boundaries. With BodyWHealth, I will enjoy its abundant riches forever!

Today, I understand the physical basis of health and happiness better than ever before. I am still a physician and a scientist, and as such my new understanding is grounded firmly in fact. Scientists don't know everything yet, and that's exciting. But there is a whole lot that we do know, and the emerging knowledge is thrilling. It tells me that there is irrefutable evidence that our WHealth is in our own hands. For me, this is an enthralling and weighty realization.

I hope that the ideas in this book revolutionize your life the way they revolutionized mine. Every single one of us is entitled to the abundant riches of BodyWHealth. To get you there, this book describes the science behind WHealth and outlines a simple pathway to achieve it. From the ah-ha moment of knowing you deserve it to the incredibly gratifying moment of knowing you've attained it, I know it works. *Please join me on this magnificent journey to BodyWHealth!*

WHAT IS BODYWHEALTH?

Before we start the journey, let's evaluate the prize: *Abundant WHealth!*

That's so easy to say, yet so hard to describe. You know when you have it, and you know when you don't. You recognize when somebody else has it, and you recognize when they don't. Those who have it glow. They have a bounce and resilience in their gait and their lives. They radiate optimism, hope, and purpose, and give to the world with seemingly endless generosity.

Let me start by asking you a few questions:

Are you the best you that you could possibly be?

Do you have energy for life, every day?

Do you wake each morning feeling rested, inspired for the day ahead?

Do you look in the mirror and like what you see, even when you're naked?

Are you running your life instead of your life running you?

Are you doing what you love, and do you love what you're doing?

Are you loved, and do you love?

Do you know your value to the world?

Do you have a purpose beyond yourself?

Are you handsomely rewarded for your contributions to the world?

When you can answer *all* of these questions with an emphatic, confident "YES," then you have BodyWHealth.

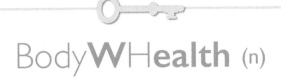

BodyWHealth (n)

A personal growth strategy that optimizes your biology to achieve abundance. Based on evolutionary principles and scientific evidence, BodyWHealth is a proven pathway to health, happiness and prosperity.

Two profound insights are fundamental to BodyWHealth.

The first is that the pace of our social and technological evolution has vastly outstripped our physiological evolution. We are not biologically adapted to the world we have created, and live in, today. To be healthy, we must live yesterday's life in today's world.

The second insight is that each of us will achieve BodyWHealth only when we *believe* that we deserve it. Most of us believe that bountiful health, happiness, and prosperity are attainable only by a fortunate minority. This is *false*. The abundant riches of WHealth are available to each of us, but only if we believe—truly *believe*—that we can attain them.

THE (R)EVOLUTIONARY GAP

Modern men and women suffer the consequences of an evolutionary gap that impairs our health and happiness. Social and technological advances have rapidly outstripped our biology. To have BodyWHealth, we must live yesterday's behaviors in today's world!

Biological adaptation is a slow process. The earliest signs of life on earth were simple single-celled organisms called prokaryotes, thought to have originated about 4.6 billion years ago. Via a very slow process, they evolved to become more complicated single-cell organisms called eukaryotes. This journey took roughly 1.5 billion years. Another billion years later, the first multicellular organisms appeared. This brings us to a point on the timeline of history about 1 billion years ago. Yes, still *billion*, with a "B."

It took another 400 million years before we could recognize these multicellular organisms as animals; the very first appeared 600 million years ago. Now the evolutionary clock starts to speed up (but it's still very slow by modern standards). The first mammals appeared 200 million years ago. Primates eventually appeared some 60 million years ago, but they took their time before they looked anything like we do. The first upright (bipedal) primates made an entrance 2.5 million years ago. That's probably further in our rearview mirror than most of us can imagine!

Finally, 200,000 years ago, *homo sapiens* (humans) stepped out of the shadows.

Since then, our biological evolution has been largely insignificant (although we still can't explain why we have an appendix). Instead, social and technological evolution has streaked ahead. Using their recently evolved cerebral cortex (the huge outermost layer of our brain that empowers us with thought and reason), our early ancestors began to master simple tools and took control of fire. It took us most of the last 200,000 years to progress toward a milestone that we all take for granted today: the discovery of electricity (almost three centuries ago).

At a dizzying, super-exponential pace, we then produced the telephone (1870s), automobiles (1890s), television (late 1920s), computers (1960s), and personal computers (1980). Two decades ago, we developed the seemingly indispensable mobile phone. Each of these quantum leaps alone transformed our lives. Collectively, they have propelled us into an era unimaginable to our grandparents, and clearly unanticipated by Mother Nature!

No species could adapt fast enough to make the biological adjustments necessary to match this technological revolution and its impact on human society. As a result, we are now facing a massive (R)evolutionary Gap with highly significant consequences.

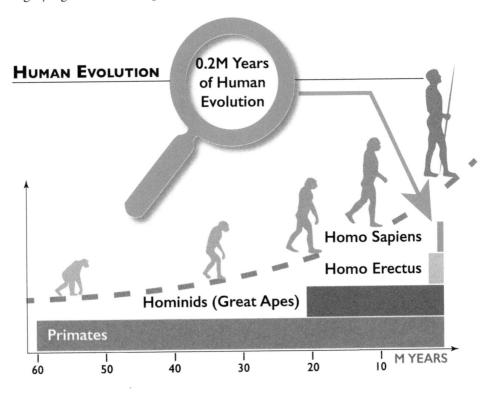

TECHNOLOGICAL AND SOCIETAL VS. PHYSICAL EVOLUTION

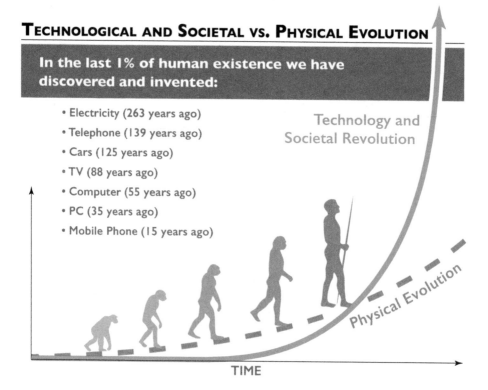

In the last 1% of human existence we have discovered and invented:

- Electricity (263 years ago)
- Telephone (139 years ago)
- Cars (125 years ago)
- TV (88 years ago)
- Computer (55 years ago)
- PC (35 years ago)
- Mobile Phone (15 years ago)

Technology and Societal Revolution

Physical Evolution

TIME

Yesterday, we were hunter-gatherers. We roamed the plains, valleys, and highlands of the planet, focusing solely on survival. We had to exercise to live. We either ate dinner or were eaten by something bigger, faster, and hungrier than ourselves. We ran to catch, and we ran to escape. We carried children, possessions, and primitive weapons in our arms and on our backs. We ate a mixed diet of unprocessed, natural foods. We were active during daylight, and we slept at night.

Fast-forward (in evolutionary terms) 200,000 years to the present. Today, we live a largely sedentary life. Exercise is voluntary for the vast majority of us. Technology makes even manual labor easier—ask any weekend warrior about our obsession with power tools. Our diets are largely processed, and food is in relative abundance (over the past twenty years in the USA, for example, portion sizes have doubled). Due to our mastery of electricity and the emergence of digital and electronic communication and entertainment, we now stay up late into the night. Our quantity and quality of sleep has deteriorated significantly.

These changes are highly prevalent in developed countries, and the "developing" world is not far behind.

And then there is *stress!* It's hard to know how our average daily stress levels compare to our ancestors, who fled for their lives from saber-toothed tigers and woolly mammoths. Certainly, though, the modern version is more intrusive and more impactful in the developed world than it is in simple agrarian cultures. It is a prominent part of our environment that we appear physiologically unprepared for.

Most of us eat processed food in excess, sit at desks or in cars or on couches and recliners all day, work too hard, and sleep too little. We are out of harmony with our physical purpose. The consequences are dire: disease, decay, and pervasive sadness.

This is the root of the BodyWHealth solution. Nature built us an exquisite body with an intricate design, including the most advanced of animal brains. We were designed to eat a natural diet, to run, to defend ourselves, to love, and to sleep. That's what we are still designed for today. When we do those things, all is well, and we are rewarded with abundant WHealth. This book explains how we unlock physical WHealth from deep within our physical being. This is the foundation on which we then build emotional WHealth. Prosperity follows. Together, these elements form the abundant WHealth that should be our common and individual goals as WHealth Seekers.

PRIMAL BALANCE

To understand this fundamental discord between our biology and our lifestyles, we need to pause to learn a little more about a critical biological balance that maintains our physical health.

There is a chemical battle that is going on in your body, even as you read this. It's a brilliant, complex drama with many characters, each with their own specific role and function. The body is a dynamic, living system comprised of millions of cells organized into working units. Just like us, these cells don't live forever. Nature has evolved an elaborate system to remove old and dead cells and replace them with new and healthy ones. Every bodily tissue is constantly being refreshed. Even bone, which seems solid, is continually being broken down and rebuilt. To achieve this process, your body has two teams that work in perfect harmony, together playing a critical role in your health. One team is responsible for breaking down old, broken, or defective tissue. The other team is responsible for growth and repair of healthy new tissue.

In the scientific community, the chemical characters I'm referring to are known as *cytokines*. They are small proteins, and they give commands to the immune cells involved with the inflammatory process. There are several cytokines on the "destroyer" team that break down tissue; they are known as *pro-inflammatory cytokines* because they invoke inflammation. The best-known pro-inflammatory cytokine is *Interleukin 6 (IL6)*. Similarly, there are several cytokines on the "builder" team that rebuild tissue. It won't surprise you to know that they are known as *anti-inflammatory cytokines* due to their role in suppressing inflammation. Their most famous member is probably *Interleukin 10 (IL10)*. In addition to overseeing the repair and reconstruction processes, the anti-inflammatory cytokines also have superiority in the chain of command, and can order the pro-inflammatory cytokine team to stop its work.

The prevailing direction of the body is decay. You know this from observing human aging. If the body is left alone, degeneration occurs. Ask anybody who has been immobilized in a cast or confined to a bed for any period of time. They experience rapid loss of muscle. It's true: "Use it or lose it." This is because, in adults, the pro-inflammatory cytokines become the dominant force by default. If left unchecked, this army causes atrophy of your working parts, leading to degeneration and aging.

Fortunately, we don't only have the pro-inflammatory cytokines. We also have the anti-inflammatory cytokines, and they work with and against their pro-inflammatory counterparts to keep us young and healthy. They do two things: with one hand, they stop the destructive work of the pro-inflammatory cytokines (they literally switch them off); and with the other hand, they lead the construction and repair crews. Certainly, we need both teams. But to stay young and healthy, we need to be sure that the anti-inflammatory cytokines are always the most active!

When you were a child, the anti-inflammatory cytokines dominated no matter what you did. They hurried around your body instructing your cells to reproduce. That's why you grew into the fine adult specimen you are today. Over your lifetime, however, the pro-inflammatory cytokines will start to get the upper hand and the natural process of aging will take over. As you've heard too many people say, "It's all downhill from here!" And in the absence of deliberate action on your part, that is true. With the pro-inflammatory cytokines dominant, you have more cells being broken down and removed than you have new cells being produced. Slowly but steadily, your tissues weaken and decay. Sounds gross, right? To make matters worse, long-term stress has been shown to augment the effect of the inflammatory army. Smoking and body fat, especially visceral body fat (that's the fat on your belly and around your internal organs), also increase the dominance of the pro-inflammatory cytokines. That's when you not only lose your BodyWHealth, but you start suffering from disease. Diabetes, heart disease, and even cancer thrive under these pro-inflammatory conditions.

> ## In the absence of deliberate action on your part, you are destined for degeneration and decay!

But there is fantastic news: Exercise drives the anti-inflammatory cytokines!

Actually, the first thing that happens after a serious bout of exercise is mobilization of the pro-inflammatory cytokines. We want this, because the (desirable) stress of exercise almost invariably results in minor damage to healthy tissues. We need those pro-inflammatory cytokines to bring the immune cells in to break down and clear damaged tissue. But here is the magic! After a short time, the anti-inflammatory cytokines are also mobilized. In fact, the predominant, lasting benefit of exercise is that the anti-inflammatory cytokines jump into action. The first thing they do is to switch off the pro-inflammatory cytokines, who would otherwise continue their energetic efforts to the point of harm. Instead, IL10 and her army stop the demolition gangs. They call loudly for reconstruction to start. Immune cells bring in healthy new material to rebuild, and get to work repairing damaged tissue. The (healthy) stress of regular exercise prevents long-term domination of the pro-inflammatory cytokines. It keeps you young and healthy.

This is the central thesis of BodyWHealth: The combination of regular exercise and limiting the volume of visceral body fat helps your anti-inflammatory cytokines to dominate the cytokine balance. This makes you young. This makes you WHealthy!

ANTI-INFLAMMATORY CYTOKINES UNLOCK REJUVENATION

THE DESTROYERS	THE BUILDERS
Pro-Inflammatory Cytokines (IL6)	Anti-Inflammatory Cytokines (IL10)

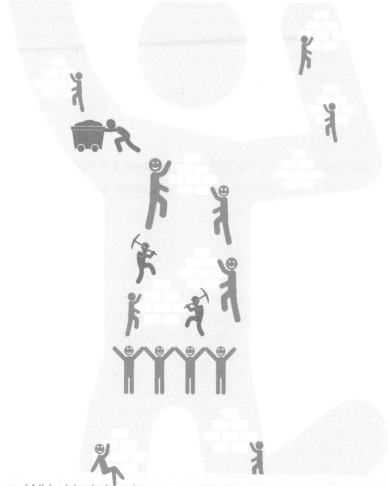

WHealthy habits (exercise, calorie balance, good sleep, and well-controlled stress) unlock the power of the anti-inflammatory cytokines to build health and youth.

INFLAMMATORY CYTOKINES DRIVE DEGENERATION AND DECAY

THE DESTROYERS
Pro-Inflammatory Cytokines (IL6)

THE BUILDERS
Anti-Inflammatory Cytokines (IL10)

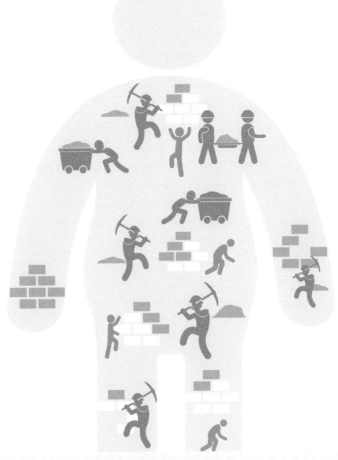

In the absence of WHealthy habits (insufficient exercise, calorie excess, poor sleep, and excessive stress), the destructive power of the inflammatory cytokines prevail, leading to degeneration, decay, and premature aging.

Let's return now to our ancestors. In their natural state, these hunter-gatherers enjoyed a balanced inflammatory system. Exercise, leanness, natural food, and plentiful sleep ensured a strong anti-inflammatory army. Their anti-inflammatory cytokines were robust and powerful. The strident voice of IL10 was heard in all the corridors and factories of the human body, commanding her cellular army to build. The prevailing mode was rejuvenation. Our ancestors died of things like accidents and infections, but not inflammatory diseases like coronary artery disease or type 2 diabetes. They had BodyWHealth.

The (R)evolutionary Gap has changed all of this. Limited (or no) exercise, proliferation of visceral fat, synthetic diets, and sleep deprivation have supercharged the pro-inflammatory cytokines. They have the upper hand. The prevailing mode is now decay and degeneration. This pro-inflammatory overload results in the distorted prevalence of coronary artery disease, type 2 diabetes, cancer, and premature death. Add stress to this toxic load, and you can see how our physical and immune resilience takes a knock...and with that, in very rapid succession, our emotional health and happiness is profoundly compromised.

YOUR HIERARCHY OF NEEDS

You will notice that I couple physical and emotional health. This is one of the most powerful BodyWHealth concepts.

Your emotional health is intimately linked to your physical condition, for several reasons. First, your emotions stem from specific areas deep within your brain. These centers are found in mammals and not in more primitive animals. For the purposes of our discussion, we will refer to this collection of specialized nerves as the "emotional brain." Just like any other part of your body, the emotional brain is a physical organ. Although it plays host to your intangible emotions, its basis is profoundly physical. Second, many of your emotions, and your mood (which is closely related), are mediated by chemicals. Again, a physical phenomenon seated deep within your body determines your emotional health.

The physical roots of mood and emotion give us tangible means to influence them for the good, toward WHealth.

Perhaps the strongest reason for me to couple physical and emotional health relates to the pioneering work of social scientists in the middle of the last century. Psychologist Abraham Maslow first published his famous "Theory of Human Motivation" in *Psychological Review* in 1943. After studying some of the world's greatest achievers and the top 1 percent of a college student population, he outlined his theory on the hierarchy of factors that motivate human behavior. He continued to expand and refine the theory throughout his career. Today, Maslow's *Hierarchy of Needs* remains a theoretical pillar of modern psychology and is widely used for both research and instruction.

Although not Maslow's original intent, the hierarchy is popularly represented as a pyramid. I, however, prefer to see it as a ladder.

As with a regular ladder, we must master the lower rungs before we can advance upward; we skip the bottom rungs at our peril. If you study the ladder carefully, you will see that mastery of the lower levels has a great deal to do with our body—our physical and emotional health. This is why I call my own philosophy and practice "BodyWHealth." It is only through sustained investment in our Body that we can attain the WHealth found at higher functional levels.

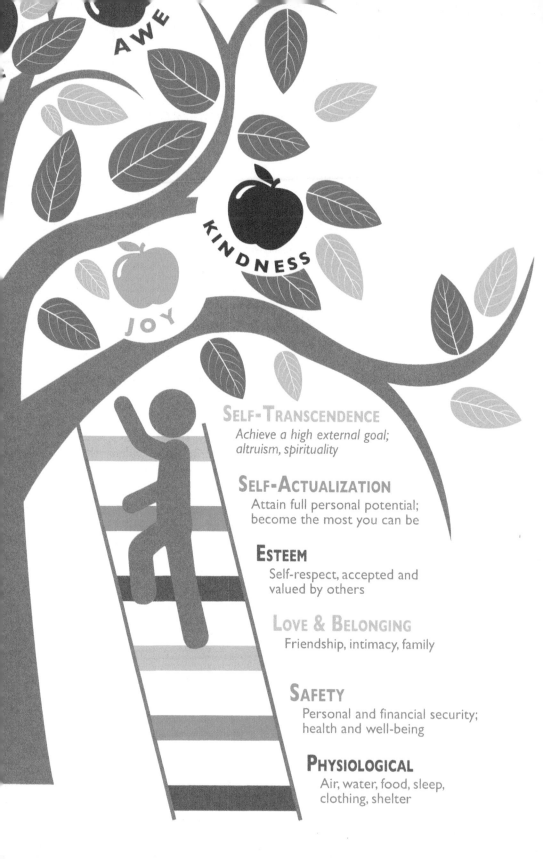

AWE

KINDNESS

JOY

SELF-TRANSCENDENCE
Achieve a high external goal; altruism, spirituality

SELF-ACTUALIZATION
Attain full personal potential; become the most you can be

ESTEEM
Self-respect, accepted and valued by others

LOVE & BELONGING
Friendship, intimacy, family

SAFETY
Personal and financial security; health and well-being

PHYSIOLOGICAL
Air, water, food, sleep, clothing, shelter

Like any model, Maslow's Hierarchy of Needs is an imperfect embodiment of life; in particular, it lacks robust translation across diverse global cultures. Still, it has sufficient accuracy for us to use it as a framework to guide our own efforts and judge our progress.

The first step of the ladder describes our need for the most basic life-sustaining physical elements: air, water, food, sleep, clothing, and shelter. Until we have these, we can't contemplate the next level, which includes our need for personal and financial security. This grouping, described as "safety needs" by Maslow, includes physical health and well-being. Having satisfied our basic physical requirements, we can progress to the third level, where we begin to address our emotional needs with family, intimacy, and friendship. The fourth level motivates us to address our self-esteem as we search for recognition and respect, initially from others and ultimately from ourselves. Maslow suggests that these four steps comprise the essential framework for successful life, and intimates that the subsequent "growth" steps take us beyond simply living to "self-actualization" and ultimately "self-transcendence." He asserts that mastery of the first four stages is required before you can reach the highest rungs.

It is important for WHealth Seekers to know two things about this model. First, although it appears to be a logical modular progression, it isn't. We are driven by needs at several levels at any one point in time. One level tends to dominate, and that is where we spend most of our time and energy. Second, we don't only move upward. As we live our lives, we go up and down the ladder. Events, often beyond our control, can bump us down to lower levels. For example, a financial disaster or professional setback can rob us of both the self-confidence of level four and the financial security of level two. We must drop back down the ladder to secure those needs before we can again aspire to the riches at the top.

One of the problems with setbacks, which can be frequently recurring events, is the way we respond. We often neglect our bodies at exactly the time we should be focusing on our physical health. All too often, we slump into an unhealthy pile on the couch, burying our sadness in calories and neglecting exercise. Or, we stop eating, neglecting our physical condition with calorie restriction. Or, in an attempt to claw our way back up the ladder, we overwork. And when we overwork, we overeat, under-exercise, and lose sleep. We trigger a vicious cycle in which the pro-inflammatory cytokines triumph and erode our BodyWHealth, sometimes with catastrophic results.

Each of us has our own individual ladder. It is the way we access fruit in the orchard of life. We can reach low-hanging fruit by using the lowest rungs of our ladder. But the sweetest fruit is at the top of the trees. We have to master our ladder to consistently feast on life's greatest riches.

THE POWER OF BELIEF

There is one more potent phenomenon we as WHealth Seekers need to contemplate before we start our journey. Its origins are multifactorial, in part the consequences of the (R)evolutionary Gap and the gravitational downward force we experience on Maslow's ladder.

The desperately sad reality is that we no longer believe that we deserve youth, health, and happiness. We consider these to be elusive privileges, like material wealth, that are granted to only a tiny minority. We believe that decay and degeneration are the prevailing order, and we sit there waiting for those forces to creep inevitably through our bodies. I am convinced that this is the single biggest challenge to BodyWHealth, and to individual and societal health and happiness. If you believe that you are doomed to decay, I guarantee that this will be your fate. If you believe that you do not deserve WHealth, you simply will not have it.

On the other hand, if you believe that you deserve the abundant riches of youth, health, and happiness, you will enjoy them! The key to success is to have your mind lead your body. This is the great secret of BodyWHealth.

READER'S GUIDE TO *BodyWHealth*

This book outlines the path to BodyWHealth. Insight into the cytokine battle will give you immense power. You no longer have to watch the battle as a passive, aging onlooker. You can *command* the armies, and you will be rewarded with rejuvenation, youth, and health!

You will learn that BodyWHealth is the best investment you can make. It takes hard work to sustain the habits required to achieve physical health and to advance your journey up Maslow's ladder. It takes great courage to pursue emotional development at the next level. But the rewards are rich. At the highest levels in the hierarchy of life, we engage in altruism: a selfless, mindful, purposeful generosity of being. Compelling scientific data continue to emerge describing the abundant benefits of this state.

This book has three main sections that will build your knowledge and guide you on your journey to abundant WHealth. This is your roadmap to health, happiness, and prosperity.

The first section, "The Physical Foundation," will revolutionize your insight into the value of physical WHealth. Understanding the science of your body in its evolutionary context will inspire you to WHealthy actions. You will build a physical foundation that honors your biological design and purpose. In particular, you will learn about the first three Keys to physical WHealth:

Key #1:   Step Up
Key #2:   Count Calories
Key #3:   Sleep Right

In the second section, we will explore "The Enabling Mindsets." As the name suggests, these powerful mindsets foster real, lasting change, and will help you to move from aspiration to application of the first three Keys. The mindsets are captured in the fourth and fifth Keys:

Key #4:   Conquer Excuses
Key #5:   BELIEVE

You will want to read this section carefully, perhaps more than once. If you embrace it, new insight into the power of belief will transform your life.

The 7 Keys of Body**WH**ealth

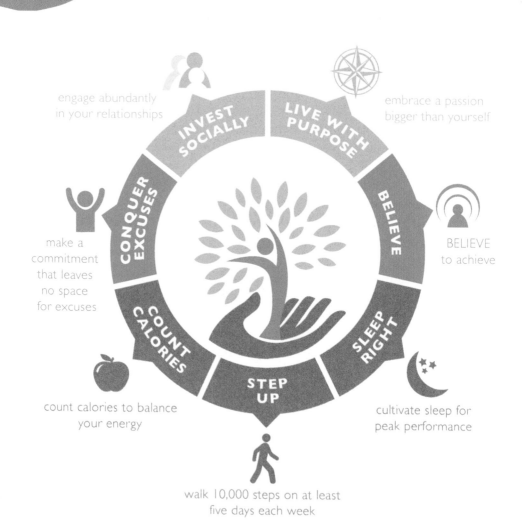

engage abundantly
in your relationships

embrace a passion
bigger than yourself

INVEST SOCIALLY

LIVE WITH PURPOSE

CONQUER EXCUSES

BELIEVE

make a
commitment
that leaves
no space
for excuses

BELIEVE
to achieve

COUNT CALORIES

SLEEP RIGHT

STEP UP

count calories to balance
your energy

cultivate sleep for
peak performance

walk 10,000 steps on at least
five days each week

The final section, "Beyond Physical WHealth," describes your payoff. You unlock physical WHealth, using the first five Keys, in order to enjoy emotional WHealth and prosperity. You will learn that these are not random gifts for a lucky few. Your path will be illuminated by the final two Keys to emotional WHealth:

Key #6:   **Invest Socially**
Key #7:   **Live with Purpose**

Insight into the empowering science of emotional WHealth, which starts deep within you, will drive you toward your ultimate goal—prosperity— where you will be recognized and rewarded for the value you bring to the world. Above all others, this insight will convince you that your WHealth truly is in *your* hands.

You'll notice as you work your way through this book that I use the term "we" quite frequently, and to describe two different groups. I am here to link you as a WHealth Seeker with the science of BodyWHealth. Sometimes I use "we" to include myself with you in the WHealth-seeking community of people who want health, happiness, and prosperity for life. At other times I use "we" to include myself in the scientific community that has conducted and is continuing to conduct powerful research to support the WHealth concepts.

I don't pretend to have all the answers, but I do know a simple recipe that works, because it worked for me. I will share with you the pathway and the science behind it. Through knowledge comes insight, and with insight you will have power: the power to achieve physical and emotional WHealth and prosperity.

If you already have BodyWHealth, congratulations! I believe that you will still find value in this book. Having achieved BodyWHealth, I continue to work each day to preserve and enhance it, and I believe that there will be insights and ideas here to help you preserve and enhance your BodyWHealth, too.

Please join the online community at www.BodyWHealth.org. There, you have access to exclusive online content that will enhance your journey as a WHealth Seeker. You will also find ways to connect with other WHealth Seekers, to share stories and experiences along the way.

CALL TO ACTION

There are two reasons why I can assure you that the BodyWHealth formula works.

First, I have followed it personally, and it has transformed my life!

Second, and perhaps even more importantly, over the past fifteen years leading scientists have conducted a series of landmark studies. This research systematically evaluated the role that lifestyle plays in causing (or preventing) disease and premature death. The combined studies evaluated almost half a million human subjects—an extraordinary feat of observation. The data provide irrefutable scientific proof of the massive impact that lifestyle modification, including exercise, weight reduction, and improved sleep, has on your health; the data show a 90 percent reduction in heart attack, a 91 percent reduction in type 2 diabetes, and a 50 percent reduction in stroke.

The prize of physical health should be sufficient to motivate you to read further and to implement the simple BodyWHealth formula into your daily life. Add to this the emotional WHealth that you will build on top of this physical platform, and the case is irresistible!

You *can* live the life you were designed for! When you understand the science and the evolutionary context, you can build the physical foundation for your health and happiness. If you honor your primal design and constructively "manage" your mental and emotional disposition, you absolutely can attain WHealth. If you believe—truly *believe*—that you deserve it, then the abundant riches of BodyWHealth will be yours. Your WHealth is in *your* hands!

THE
PHYSICAL
FOUNDATION

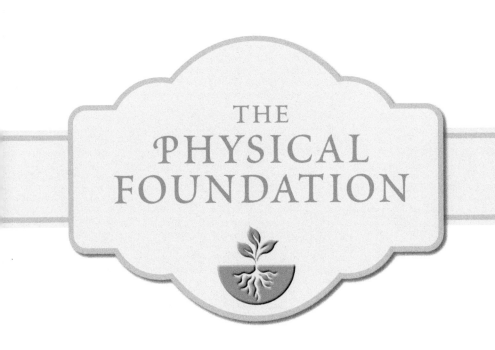

Whereas the destination is majestic, the start of the journey is imminently practical.

Our ultimate WHealth interest is a colorful assortment of glorious riches including youth, health, happiness, fulfillment, mindfulness, self-competence, self-confidence, self-determination, selflessness, and self-actualization. It borders on the spiritual, as captured in Maslow's "self-transcendence" terminology.

In contrast, the early steps of the WHealth Seeker's journey are simple and pragmatic. Many of us consider the body to be only a *physical* vehicle—the arms and legs that move us through our day—but it goes well beyond that. It also comprises the five senses that give us awareness, the being that enables love, and the brain that helps us to think and dream. Every one of these functions requires a healthy chemical foundation and the energy to drive it.

As you start to work on the bodily basics, know that you are building your intangible future. The physical foundation is not simply a stage that starts the journey. It's not something you graduate from to move toward higher things. Instead, the physical foundation *becomes* your journey. The power of BodyWHealth is this intimate, enduring link between the Body and WHealth. It is a simple road to glorious riches.

There are many things you must do to be healthy. You must brush your teeth, see your doctor for regular checkups, screen yourself for common and serious health threats, immunize yourself against infectious diseases, protect yourself from sun damage…and the list goes on. But for our purposes here, we will focus on four aspects of our biology: three that work *for* us, namely exercise, calorie balance, and sleep; and one that conspires *against* us, stress.

There is a very simple reason why these four are the central themes of physical health: Above all other factors, they have an immense impact on the inflammatory cytokine balance, and hence on systemic (whole-body) inflammation. If we get them wrong, we slide down the default pathway of degeneration and decay. If we get them right, we tip our biological balance into a more youthful state: BodyWHealth.

Please stay in close contact with your medical team as you make major lifestyle changes. If you have been inactive for some time and are out of shape, it's probably a good idea to see your doctor before you change your exercise and dietary habits. And, if in doubt at any subsequent time about your body's condition, check back in with your doctor. You have to be healthy to be WHealthy!

KEY #1: STEP UP

Walk 10,000 steps on at least five days each week.

A sedentary life has become a core feature of modern society. Many people sit for long hours at desks at work, and then go home exhausted to collapse in front of the television. I'm sure that many of you reading this chapter are just like I was, spending your day working hard mentally, but stationary physically. And this is where BodyWHealth's first Key comes into play.

A few years ago, the British Medical Journal published research[1] that quantified the impact of a sedentary lifestyle on our health. Aggregating the data from several studies on the same topic, the authors concluded that "sedentary behaviors are accounting for between 1.4 and 2.0 years of life expectancy." Breaking this down further, the data show that if you are able to limit sitting to less than three hours per day, you could increase your life expectancy by two years. Similarly, limiting television-watching to less than two hours per day should increase your life expectancy by 1.4 years.

The most current research concludes emphatically that an aerobic activity base of 10,000 steps on at least five days each week is *the way* to restore our natural physiology. This is the first step toward rejuvenation. If you desire WHealth, you have no choice.

When we talk about a healthy body, we essentially mean a body that is doing what we want it to, when we want it to, and seeing some evidence that it's going to be doing this for some time. Right? And so, we should ask: What exactly was our body designed to do? And to answer this, we need to remember our origins and the time scale we as human beings are living on.

First, what were we designed to do? As a biologist, I can tell you that we were designed to build, nurture, and propagate our species. In simple terms, we were made to have children and to ensure that they survive to have their own children. In order to do that, we have to compete for a mate, be attractive to a mate, mate with our mate, give birth to our children, feed them, fight off adversaries who want to eat our lunch (or eat us for lunch!), and live long enough to protect our children until they can make use of their own fertility. It may not sound very elegant, but it's true. In order to do all of this, we need to be fit and strong. To be fit and strong, we need to be constantly exercising.

So, that's what we were designed to do, and for our bodies to be healthy and happy, that's what we as WHealth Seekers *must* do! Mother Nature understands this. In her design, she ensured that exercise triggers an addictive cascade of chemical changes within our body, which together drive WHealth.

THE BIOLOGICAL CONSEQUENCES OF EXERCISE

We often talk about the *benefits* of exercise. I prefer to use the word *consequences* because I want you to know that your decision to exercise (or not) has a profound impact in your life. There are real consequences either way. If you exercise, you invoke Mother Nature's powers of rejuvenation. If you do not, you expressly agree to the default rule of relentless degeneration and decay.

Two streams of scientific research inform our knowledge about the vital role of exercise as a foundation of WHealth. With the authority of retrospect, we are able to view these two critical streams that started independently, ran in parallel for a while, and then converged to give us some magical answers about exercise and health.

The first stream of research focused on understanding the underlying cause of premature death and suffering in the developed world. As we searched for explanations for major diseases and events like heart attacks, strokes, type 2 diabetes, obesity, high blood pressure, cancer, and neurodegenerative diseases like dementia and Alzheimer's disease, we started to find the dirty fingerprints of inflammation. In response, scientists doubled their efforts to understand the elaborate complexity of inflammation, particularly in these diseased states. We don't have definitive, crystal-clear answers yet, but it's fair to say that a scientific consensus is emerging that a common theme— perhaps *the* common theme among many of these age-linked, degenerative conditions—is chronic inflammatory overload.

And guess what? The more our societies have "developed," the more we have seen these diseases surge, claiming and maiming our loved ones prematurely.

It is no coincidence that at the same time, these developing societies have become increasingly inactive, predominantly sedentary in habit.

Our ancestors exercised to live. Exercise was not a separate activity; it was an integral part of their lives. As we "modernized" through the Industrial Revolution, we began to pride ourselves on inactivity. We celebrated innovations, like the car and the computer, that reduced our physical burden. Not so long ago, scientists started to take note of a part of our lives that had become separated from the mainstream and turned into an optional activity for those who liked it. In what became the second pivotal stream of research, we learned about the recreational role of exercise and soon began exploring its value to our health, focusing initially on the major biological systems involved: the heart, the lungs, and the muscles. As our insight grew with more probing technology, we started to study what was happening at a chemical and subsequently genetic level.

The intriguing part of this second stream of research is that we began to notice how the pro- and anti-inflammatory cytokines seemed to play a major role in exercise. When we first discovered the presence of inflammation, we explained it by saying that exercise was damaging muscles, and the chemicals that leaked out of those damaged muscle cells summoned the inflammatory armies to repair them. What blew our minds as the research advanced was the discovery that exercise provokes an inflammatory response even without muscle damage!

So, we went back to the drawing board to understand the reason for post-exercise inflammation. Here is what we found: During or immediately after a single bout of intense exercise in generally sedentary people, their bodies were inundated with pro-inflammatory chemicals. We found cytokines in their blood and muscles that provoke inflammation. In contrast, when we studied athletes who were accustomed to regular, sustained exercise, we found remarkably little inflammation. The predominant chemicals in their blood were anti-inflammatory. It appeared that the stress of acute, occasional exercise drove inflammation but that regular exercise suppressed it.

Previously, we had advocated exercise for health only because of its propensity to reduce weight. We knew that exercise increased metabolic demand for energy. We also knew that, if we kept incoming dietary energy (food) constant, the increased demands of exercise had the body reaching into fat stores to meet its energy requirements. If the body's energy demands regularly exceeded dietary intake, we were able to drive weight loss. We knew that obesity was dangerous, so we recommended exercise plus calorie restriction to help patients lose weight.

Suddenly, the two major research streams began to converge, and we realized we had stumbled upon a health gold mine. In one laboratory we were showing how systemic inflammation was central to major disease in the developed world. In the laboratory next door, we were demonstrating how long-term exercise reduced systemic inflammation. Bingo! We started to realize how our heroic efforts to reduce the physical burden of the human race had inadvertently induced an epidemic of degenerative disease with dire personal consequences. More importantly, we began to appreciate the full therapeutic potential of exercise!

Even as we got excited about the full potential of exercise, though, we still needed to understand and explain this strange phenomenon where a single bout of exercise *induced* systemic inflammation, but regular exercise *reduced* it.

THE BATTLE TO CONTROL YOUR INFLAMMATORY DESTINY

Inflammation is part of a complex biological response of the human body to dangerous invasions (like infections and chemical irritants) and the detection of damaged or defective tissue (including cancer cells). Our body mounts an immune response in order to attack and remove the foreign invader or defective cell, to clean up the debris, and ultimately to initiate processes that restore and rejuvenate the affected tissues and organs. As opposed to adaptive immunity where we develop antibodies to fight specific infectious agents (like what comes from an immunization shot you get from your doctor), inflammation is non-specific in its approach; the same ferocious army of pro-inflammatory cytokines is unleashed in response to a wide range of different stimuli. As you can imagine, inflammation is a dangerous weapon (or arsenal, rather, because there is an entire range of weapons in it), and so it must be tightly regulated. Unopposed, inflammation would result in far-reaching destruction of the host (that's you!). To protect against this, Mother Nature developed an equally complex system to limit, and even reverse, inflammation: the anti-inflammatory cytokines. Together, these two complementary armies are known as the inflammatory system.

Inflammation is a coordinated response to a perceived threat in which your body orchestrates the work of immune cells and alters the functioning of blood vessels. The initial response is instantaneous and happens at the site at which the threat is detected. Your body immediately changes the permeability of your tiny blood vessels to allow white blood cells to leak into surrounding tissue. If you picture the little bump that swells up quickly around a mosquito bite, you'll understand this leaky blood vessel phenomenon. Your white blood cells are initial responders. Together with other local tissues, they release powerful chemicals that alert the rest of the body to the threat. Your body responds by sending patrolling inflammatory armies into the hot spot to get on with the destruction and then healing.

The demolition squad of pro-inflammatory cytokines, comprising several lines of enthusiastic immune cells, is the first to arrive. Summoned by a swarm of chemical messengers, they get on with the important roles of destruction and removal. They attack the invaders or defective cells and break them down into little pieces before ingesting them and carrying them off to various biological dumping sites. A great deal of research has focused attention on the chemical mediators of this destructive response, and we have a long list of chemicals with exotic names that participate (such as *histamine, interferon gamma,* interleukins, *leukotrienes, tumor necrosis factor, prostaglandins,* and *nitric oxide*). They are broadly known as pro-inflammatory mediators, led by IL6.

Soon after the initial response of the pro-inflammatory cytokines, the body activates the anti-inflammatory cytokines with two separate orders. First, they must limit the "damage" caused by the pro-inflammatory cytokines, whose enthusiasm and diligence would otherwise cost us dearly. Second, they must initiate the rebuilding process. Again, a long list of chemical messengers is involved in these anti-inflammatory processes (such as interleukins, *lipoxins, resolvins, protectins,* and a number of molecules that antagonize or block the pro-inflammatory messengers). They are broadly known as anti-inflammatory mediators, led by IL10.

The anti-inflammatory cytokines usually settle the inflammation and repair the damage caused by the initial threat. In some cases, though— and you'll see that it becomes extremely relevant for our health—the pro-inflammatory cytokines remain dominant. This results in long-term systemic inflammation.

GENERAL INFLAMMATORY RESPONSE

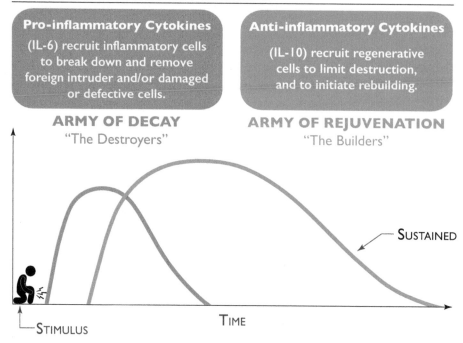

Pro-inflammatory Cytokines

(IL-6) recruit inflammatory cells to break down and remove foreign intruder and/or damaged or defective cells.

Anti-inflammatory Cytokines

(IL-10) recruit regenerative cells to limit destruction, and to initiate rebuilding.

ARMY OF DECAY
"The Destroyers"

ARMY OF REJUVENATION
"The Builders"

SUSTAINED

TIME

STIMULUS

TIPPING THE CYTOKINE BALANCE IN YOUR FAVOR

For centuries, athletes have recognized how muscle growth happens after training with intensity sufficient to take a muscle to its limit. Early exercise physiologists taught us that overloading muscles resulted in micro-tears to those muscles and their supporting structures, and that the resulting healing process provided the strength gains sought by athletes. By now you know that IL6 and the pro-inflammatory team are the first to arrive at such micro-tear injury sites.

But what you might not know is that the behavior of IL6, the leader of the pro-inflammatory cytokines, varies by exercise type. Resistance training, like lifting weights, induces a rapid peak within about four hours and a rapid decline over the subsequent twenty-four hours. In contrast, in aerobic training, like moderate-intensity running, levels of IL6 peak at around twelve hours (and sometimes as late as twenty-four hours) after exercise, followed by a gradual decline. At first, this might make you think that you should avoid aerobic exercise to avoid such a prolonged pro-inflammatory surge.

But there's more to the story! In order to balance the enthusiasm of IL6 and other pro-inflammatory cytokines, the body mobilizes the anti-inflammatory armies. The voice of IL10 starts the work that both curtails the damage of the demolition squads and recruits the reconstruction teams. Powerful forces of repair and rejuvenation are unleashed to rebuild muscle architecture. The anti-inflammatory cytokines must linger to balance the sustained inflammatory response to aerobic exercise—and we as WHealth Seekers want to encourage those anti-inflammatory cytokines to stick around as long as possible. This enduring anti-inflammatory presence is thought to be one of the reasons for the long-term health benefits of prolonged moderate-intensity exercise.

Remember how excited scientists were when we discovered that even moderate exercise that did not cause muscle damage triggered IL6 and the surge of pro-inflammatory cytokines? In the absence of micro-trauma, with no evidence of tissue that needs to be broken down and rebuilt, the body still triggers the pro-inflammatory cascade...and, more importantly, the resulting anti-inflammatory cascade. This is the magic of exercise and the fundamental biology that underpins BodyWHealth's first Key! Exercise

INFLAMMATORY RESPONSE TO EXERCISE

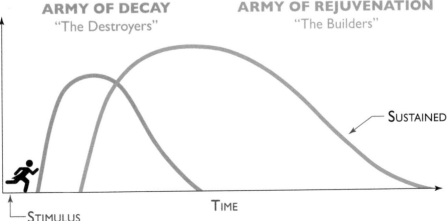

Pro-inflammatory Cytokines

(IL-6) recruit inflammatory cells to break down and remove foreign intruder and/or damaged or defective cells.

Anti-inflammatory Cytokines

(IL-10) recruit regenerative cells to limit destruction, and to initiate rebuilding.

ARMY OF DECAY
"The Destroyers"

ARMY OF REJUVENATION
"The Builders"

SUSTAINED

TIME

STIMULUS

triggers the inflammatory system, period, with far-reaching benefits. In particular, regular exercise results in sustained elevations in IL10 and the anti-inflammatory cytokines. Under their guidance, the cellular elements of our inflammatory system are predominantly engaged in building and repair. The result is rejuvenation, youth, and health.

It probably doesn't surprise you to see that the schematic for the inflammatory response to exercise is identical to the schematic showing general inflammation. In particular, you will notice the enduring response of the anti-inflammatory cytokines to pro-inflammatory stimuli. With regular exercise, you superimpose consecutive waves of rejuvenation, driving immense health benefits.

Regular exercise also stimulates the body to improve peripheral circulation. In order to better supply working muscles with nutrients and remove their waste, the body augments the quantity and volume of peripheral blood vessels. This enhanced circulatory system becomes the grand scheme of highways for the inflammatory army, enabling both the pro- and the anti-inflammatory cytokines to better patrol and service your entire body.

Our scientific appreciation of the value of muscles has progressed well beyond their role in locomotion and movement. Today we see muscles as vital organs of health, and I'm sure we've only just begun to understand their role in granting us enduring WHealth!

THE MANY BENEFITS OF EXERCISE

Regular exercise will reduce your risk of premature death. In other words, if you exercise, you have a good chance of living longer! More importantly, it will reduce your risk of dreaded diseases such as coronary artery disease, stroke, type 2 diabetes, dementia, and cancer.[2,3] So, you will live longer, be healthier, and feel better. Why? There are several reasons.

First, exercise will prolong your life. There is compelling evidence that the BodyWHealth lifestyle will result in longer life, and exercise is the cornerstone of that lifestyle.

Exercise will reduce your risk of atherosclerotic diseases. Atherosclerosis is the major underlying factor in most coronary artery disease, heart attacks, some kidney disease, and many strokes. We used to think this was a problem of lipid (fat) storage and targeted our therapy toward controlling levels of cholesterol in the blood. Now we know that exercise has a positive and independent impact on the metabolism of blood fats and lipoproteins, especially *High Density Lipoprotein (HDL)*, the "good cholesterol." More importantly, today we understand that inflammation plays a critical role in the onset, progression, and deadly catastrophes associated with atherosclerosis. In addition to favorably modifying cholesterol metabolism, the long-term anti-inflammatory benefits of exercise are recognized as core to the prevention and treatment of these devastating diseases.

Exercise will reduce your risk of type 2 diabetes. We originally believed that type 2 diabetes was a failure of the pancreas and *insulin*, the hormone it secretes, to control sugar metabolism. In this condition, the body struggles to transport sugar into working cells, leaving very high concentrations of it in the blood. Exercise stimulates cellular uptake of sugar, independent of insulin, and so we have always advocated exercise to patients with type 2 diabetes and pre-diabetes. But today we understand the destructive role of inflammation in disrupting the production of insulin by the pancreas as well as in increasing the body's sensitivity to circulating insulin. In addition to enhancing sugar uptake by cells, the long-term anti-inflammatory benefits of exercise are now recognized as core to the prevention and treatment of these severe metabolic disruptions.

Exercise will help you to control your weight. We will discuss obesity and fat metabolism in more detail in the next chapter, but I will say here that we have long recognized the role that exercise plays in increasing metabolic activity and controlling weight. Today, we understand that fat cells (especially belly fat) play an important role in driving inflammation, explaining the role of obesity as an independent cause of metabolic disease and premature death. The long-term anti-inflammatory benefits of exercise are recognized as a means of opposing the pro-inflammatory state of obesity, in addition to being a central component of any weight-reduction program.

Exercise will help your immune system to fight cancer. Exercise improves your ability to prevent and fight cancer. There is good evidence that several cancers, including colon, breast, endometrial, and lung cancers, are less prevalent in regular exercisers. Emerging evidence suggests that systemic inflammatory overload may induce genetic changes that allow normal cells to become cancerous. Inflammation also plays a role in supporting the proliferation and migration of cancer cells. Happily, regular moderate exercise has an enduring positive effect on your immune system, supporting the fight against cancerous cells. Exercise has also been shown to have a substantial positive effect on mood in people fighting cancer.

Exercise will strengthen your bones and keep you active. Unopposed, all tissues suffer at the hands of IL6 and the pro-inflammatory armies of decay. Even bone is an active tissue, with ongoing destruction and rebuilding taking place throughout life. Unless we do something to change the balance, the destructive process outweighs the rebuilding and bone mineral density declines with age. Exercise places physical stress on the bones. This is the strongest stimulus for rebuilding. Thin bones are brittle bones. They break easily, and the consequences of fractures can be devastating as you age. Exercise not only keeps the bones strong but also maintains the stability of joints and the function of nerves that facilitate balance and coordination, reducing the risk of falls. Exercise also improves joint mobility and triggers the release of natural painkillers that limit the impact of arthritis.

Finally, exercise will strengthen your mood and mental health. Exercise stimulates the release of endorphins and other hormones that improve your mood. It has also been shown to enhance intellectual function and sleep (you will see later how this is a critical element of your WHealth). Finally, there is evidence that inflammation plays a role in some of the degenerative dementias and Alzheimer's disease. There may even be a link between inflammation and depression. The long-term anti-inflammatory effects of exercise are exciting to researchers in preventing all these conditions.

Your Prescription for WHealth

Now that we better understand the chemical beauty of our design and the role that exercise plays in rejuvenation and health, let's return to our biological timeline. To fully appreciate the exercise imperative, we must recognize what has happened since our species was first designed and built. In an evolutionary nanosecond, the vast majority of us have changed from a society of physical hunter-gatherers out on the plains or mountains or beaches to a largely sedentary population. Our primary biological goal (perpetuation of our genes) has not changed, but today we use our brains more than our brawn. This (R)evolutionary Gap has created a massive problem. Our adaptive body design has not kept pace with the extraordinary rate of social and behavioral evolution we have enjoyed. No body possibly could. So, we're still living in bodies that require exercise in order to be healthy. Without exercise, we simply don't trigger the cascade of chemicals that make us healthy and happy. In fact, without exercise, we allow a whole team of destructive chemicals to prevail.

Hopefully you now accept the importance of exercise, and you're on the edge of your seat, waiting to begin your own exercise journey. But you probably still have one important question for me: "What exercise should I do?"

Here is the simplest, most powerful answer, one that I know has the capacity to transform your life: *You must walk 10,000 steps on at least five days of each week for the rest of your life!*

The results of a landmark study[4] were shared for the first time in a top-tier medical journal in April 2015. Researchers from the National Cancer Institute, the American Cancer Society, Johns Hopkins University, the Karolinska Institute, and Harvard Medical School explored data from 661,137 American and European adults over a fourteen-year period. In short, this milestone research (made possible by aggregating several massive patient databases) confirms the incremental value of exercise in reducing the risk of death. More than that, the research concluded decisively that exercise

PHYSICAL ACTIVITY REDUCES MORTALITY RISK

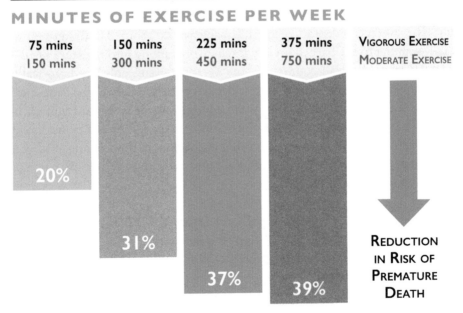

MINUTES OF EXERCISE PER WEEK

| 75 mins | 150 mins | 225 mins | 375 mins | VIGOROUS EXERCISE |
| 150 mins | 300 mins | 450 mins | 750 mins | MODERATE EXERCISE |

20%

31%

37%

39%

REDUCTION IN RISK OF PREMATURE DEATH

equivalent to 10,000 steps on at least five days each week is the optimal strategy for prime physical health.

The study, published online in the prestigious *Journal of the American Medical Association,* showed that 450 minutes of moderate exercise per week (or 225 minutes of high-intensity exercise) results in a substantial 37 percent decrease in the risk of death.[5] There is a tiny additional decrease in risk from exercising for longer periods, but the benefit appears to plateau after 450 and 225 minutes (that's 7½ and 3¾ hours) respectively. The current Physical Activity Guideline for Americans[6] of 150 minutes of moderate exercise or 75 minutes of intense exercise per week also drives a significant (but less impressive) decrease of 20 percent, over no exercise at all.

So, the magic number appears to be 450 minutes (or 7½ hours) of exercise per week. If you do the math, this equates very closely to the magic 10,000 steps on at least five days per week. This rule is important whether you're a healthy thirty-five-year-old in good shape or an aging sixty-five-year-old who hasn't exercised for twenty years.

Let's explore this 10,000-step goal a little closer. Ten thousand steps is the equivalent of five miles if you have an average stride of about 2.5 feet, and it should take you about ninety minutes if you walk a little faster than the average walking speed of three miles per hour. That adds up to 450 minutes per week. Remember, though, that this target is your goal for the entire day. The average sedentary person already walks about 2,000 steps in a day—walking to the bathroom and kitchen, or walking into the store or the cafeteria at work. It all counts. So, the average person only needs to walk an extra 8,000 *exercise* steps a day on five days of the week. Eight thousand steps are equivalent to about four miles and take about an hour if you walk at a brisk pace. If that seems like a big chunk of time, then cut it up. Walk for twenty-five minutes in the morning and again in the evening, and get up from your desk for a five-minute walk mid-morning and mid-afternoon. Easy! You've reached your goal.

If 8,000 exercise steps feel like a reach, then start with 1,000 steps (less than ten minutes), or whatever small number seems achievable. Then add 500 additional steps each week. Using this model, it would take you about fifteen weeks to reach your goal.

There are many ways to track your 10,000 steps, and I admit that as a health geek and a tech geek, I am thrilled by the host of exciting gadgets in development and at WHealth Seekers' disposal today that can help us to monitor our health and fitness, and ultimately our BodyWHealth. I call this equipment WHealthTech.

The plethora of available health-monitoring products can be confusing. I'm frequently asked, "What is the single most important health metric I should track?" I have a consistent answer: Monitor your daily activity using a step counter. That's the first step (pun intended) toward BodyWHealth. If it's the only thing you measure, you're off to a great start!

The fancy name for this type of device is *pedometer*, and they come in all shapes and sizes and prices. You can clip them to your belt, your bra, your shoelace, or your wrist. Mine is built into my smart watch, and most smartphones can also do the job perfectly. (If you'd like more information about the step counter I use, please visit my blog.) You can record your steps, beam them by satellite, compete with friends, and get really fancy. Or, you can simply look at the report at the end of the day, pat yourself on the back, and then enjoy a good night's sleep knowing you're doing a fantastic job. If you have a pedometer, use it. If you don't, get one!

Ten thousand steps is the rallying call for BodyWHealth. It delivers exactly what we need physiologically, and almost everybody can do it. It is not, however, the only exercise that will achieve the results you need. There are many alternatives, and there is good reason to experiment with more than one form of exercise. You can row, cycle, swim, jump, skip, dance, or engage in any other form of aerobic exercise. Variation will keep you mentally sharp, and using a broad range of muscle groups is beneficial to your health.

The chart below shows how several common alternatives rate against the magic 10,000-step recommendation. This table allows you to choose alternatives that stimulate an equivalent, enduring anti-inflammatory residual effect. If you're interested, you can find more expansive lists online. This will help you to mix up your exercise prescription a bit, keeping you fresh, motivated, and healthy.

There are several good online calculators that will help you estimate how many calories you will burn doing your exercise. I use the calculator built into

CALORIE BURN OF 167LB PERSON EXERCISING FOR 1 HOUR

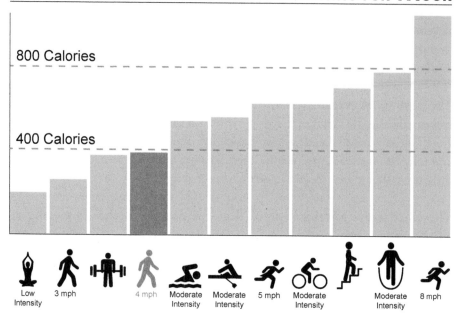

a calorie-tracking app on my mobile phone. A good calculator will adjust for three important variables that can affect your calorie-burning estimate. First is your weight. The more you weigh, the more you need to carry, and the more energy you will burn during exercise. Second, the duration of exercise is important. Your calorie burn increases in a linear fashion under most circumstances. If you double the duration of exercise, you will double your calorie burn. Finally, the type and intensity of exercise makes a big difference. Intense, high-speed running and swimming and jumping rope burn energy much faster than a slow amble in the park.

I strongly advise that you measure and log your activity every day, and every week, at least until you are sufficiently experienced to estimate it with some degree of accuracy. I did this meticulously when I started my own journey to WHealth. Today, I can dispense with the formal activity log and still be sure that I reach my exercise goals each week. It is no longer a labor. This is an important point, because the early steps in your journey can feel burdensome. But they will pass quickly. Soon, you will be in the habit of exercise and will be able to easily ensure you're getting your 10,000 steps.

Actually, you will be able to go even further than this. You will be able to estimate the number of calories you have burned in a day, both from exercise and from regular daily activities. You'll see why this is important in the next chapter. For now, focus on your steps and enjoy the journey.

I am often asked whether exercise or diet is more important for health. As you begin, which one should you focus on first? Of course, my true answer is "both," but there is absolutely no doubt in my mind that exercise comes first. An interesting research study[7] from the University of South Carolina demonstrated that body mass index and waist circumference are both more consistently associated with exercise than with diet. That's why the *first* Key to WHealth prescribes 10,000 steps and the *second* Key is about calories. So, to start, make sure that you achieve the equivalent of 10,000 steps on at least five days each week. It's a simple but powerful step on the road to BodyWHealth.

SIMPLE RECOMMENDATIONS FOR STEPPING UP

1. *See your doctor first.* Yes, I know, this is a boring reminder. But it's smart. If you're starting an exercise program, particularly if you're out of shape and have been for some time, check in with your health care provider first! And, if you are in doubt at any subsequent time about your body, check back in with your doctor. You must be healthy to be WHealthy!

2. *Start slow.* When I was younger, I always went for a run on January 1. I woke that day full of ambition and resolution. In my enthusiasm, I always ran faster than I should have. Consequently, the first week of each year was painful, and it became a strong disincentive for exercise. If you've been sedentary for a long time, you can begin by simply walking to the mailbox or once around the block. That's a great start!

3. *Build slow.* This is the same as starting slow. We've all read the fable about the tortoise and the hare. The tortoise will achieve BodyWHealth far more often than the hare. Ten years ago, I started a major reboot in my lifestyle. I started running every day, picking up the duration of each run by ten minutes per week. After two months, I had Achilles tendinitis so severe that I couldn't run without pain for several years. When I revolutionized my life with BodyWHealth, I started by walking. I built slowly, patiently working through the inevitable aches and pains as muscles, tendons, and bones all strengthened. I was patient—and it paid off big time. I'm now fifty pounds lighter and many years younger than when I started!

4. **It doesn't have to be exactly 10,000 steps.** Remember that your daily target includes regular daytime steps plus exercise steps. So, you don't need to exercise for the approximately ninety minutes required for a full 10,000 steps. Depending on how active you are during the rest of your day, you'll probably require thirty to sixty minutes of walking to hit 10,000 steps for the entire day. And if you get fewer than 10,000 steps in the beginning, that's okay.

5. **You don't have to walk.** You can walk, run, hop, skip, swim, paddle, or cycle. You can also do yoga, resistance training, and stretching. But if you're starting fresh, just aim for the primary target: 10,000 steps per day on at least five days each week. Then, if you need to work harder, find a stadium and walk up and down the steps inside. It helps if the marching band is practicing at the time (one of my personal favorites!).

6. **Break it up.** You don't have to do it all at once, and you don't need an entire new wardrobe of exercise clothes (although that may help in motivating you). You can walk the dog for twenty minutes in the morning, walk for twenty minutes over lunch, and then walk the dog again for twenty minutes in the evening, adding up to 10,000 steps total (including your regular daily activity). That makes it easy, right?

7. **Buddy up.** It's more interesting to walk and talk. Far more important, though, is the motivation of an exercise partner. When it's cold and dark when you get up in the morning to go for a walk, it helps to know that your neighbor is waiting for you at your mailbox!

8. **Consider your parking place.** This phenomenon always amazes me. Take a look at the parking lot outside any store. The parking closest to the entrance is always taken, and people are hovering, waiting for empty spots in the front, while there is plenty of space at the far end of the lot! My advice is to choose the parking spot farthest from the store entrance. Not only are there more open spots there—and not only will you avoid scratches and dings in your car because there aren't as many cars around to hit you—but it will also get you more steps! There are other similar situations you can take advantage of. Walk next to the moving walkway in the airport instead of riding on it—an especially good way to get your circulation going and your joints unfolded after long flights. Take the stairs instead of the elevator or escalator. In the words of my WHealthy son, "Exercise is an opportunity, not an inconvenience."

9. *Hold a walking meeting.* Calculate the number of hours you spend sitting in meetings or on the phone in a regular workday. Switch one meeting or phone call a day to a mobile (walking) meeting. Take your pedometer, and you'll reach your goal quicker without using up valuable personal time. When you think about it, that means you'll have your boss paying for your BodyWHealth!

10. *Have fun!* I could have put this down as all ten recommendations. You'll see this is the sign-off I use after every blog I write, too. If you can't have fun, you shouldn't be doing it. Exercise can be hard work, but it must always be fun. Listen to music. Compose poetry. Speak on the phone. Do it with a friend. Walk around the perimeter of the soccer field while your child practices. Watch surfers from the boardwalk as you run. You'll get a buzz from the endorphins, and you can enjoy intellectual and emotional pleasures, too. That's the road to WHealth!

CONCLUSION

I hope it is now very clear to you that you must reverse the devastating trend that started with the Industrial Revolution and largely eliminated exercise from your daily life. I hope you are able to stop seeing exercise as something you do just for fun, an optional extra. Instead, I hope you will regard it as an indispensible component of your life.

Exercise is the foundation of BodyWHealth. It triggers the release of the anti-inflammatory army that drives physical rejuvenation. It burns calories fast, helping you to achieve an energy balance that favors leanness, burning off excess fat that would otherwise serve as an incubator for systemic inflammation and chronic disease. It releases endorphins, protein messengers that enhance your mood, making you feel young, healthy, and happy. The more you nourish your body with these benefits, the younger you'll feel and the healthier you'll be. You will resist the natural decay of aging.

How do you start a journey of this enormous magnitude? With one step. It's that simple. And how do you start your journey to BodyWHealth? With one step. It's still that simple. Step up!

WHealth Plus

In addition to your 10,000 steps on five days of each week, I advocate that you include some resistance (strength) and flexibility training in your weekly exercise schedule. Each has unique biological benefits that drive youth and health, and variety keeps exercise fresh and fun.

THE POWER OF RESISTANCE: BUILDING STRENGTH AND REDUCING INFLAMMATION

Research over the past fifteen years has clearly demonstrated that exercise that increases muscle strength and mass has unique health benefits that add to those of aerobic exercise. In particular, resistance training promotes favorable shifts in body composition (more lean mass than fat mass), improves blood sugar control, and helps stabilize blood pressure. These are all fundamental problems in metabolic disease, and so exercise that provides these benefits is entirely desirable. Increased muscle strength has also been shown to reduce the risk of heart disease and premature death.

Like aerobic exercise, resistance training triggers the pro- and anti-inflammatory armies. In addition, muscle has a higher metabolic rate than fat. Increased muscle mass therefore speeds up your overall metabolism, particularly if you lose fat during the same period as you build up your muscles. A faster metabolism makes it easier to lose weight and to stay trim once you've lost it.

In addition to the metabolic benefits of strength training, it has skeletal benefits as well. The force that your muscles exert on your bones while working against resistance makes your bones stronger. Bone stress is a powerful stimulus and activates the anti-inflammatory cytokines in your bones, strengthening them and their supporting ligaments. Strong bones are resistant to fracture, and the resulting enhanced soft tissue strength protects joints. Similarly, having stronger bones improves balance and coordination, protecting you from injury during both exercise and daily life.

Interestingly, it turns out that handgrip strength is a good predictor of longevity. There is a reproducible, inverse relationship between grip strength and the risk of death.[8] This means that people with strong grips have a lower risk of dying than similar people with weak grips. Our strong-handshake friends are onto something!

Finally, research shows that resistance training is also associated with mental and emotional benefits. Scientists have found that regular strength training increases your energy and decreases your fatigue. Evidence is emerging for strength training's value in the management of depression and anxiety, too.

All of this is to say that there are distinct benefits to adding some resistance training into your weekly exercise schedule. If you can, I recommend that you add resistance training at least twice a week to your 10,000-step WHealthy regimen.

Strength training is a discipline filled with mystique and folklore. You will find a broad range of advice on the topic. Fads are common, and eager but unskilled advocates may put you at risk of injury. My strong recommendation is that you start your strength-training program under expert guidance. It is best to work with somebody experienced, perhaps even appropriately certified. You need a program that improves the strength, endurance, and power of your muscles without causing you harm.

There are many ways to perform resistance training. It's a good idea to experiment with a few different forms; the variation will be equally good for your body and your mind. I favor exercises that use bodyweight, free weights, and resistance bands because they minimize the risk of overload and tend to use more natural joint movements than many other methods. It is important that your program is balanced—that you exercise both sides of your body and opposing muscle groups equally. And my strong bias is to leave explosive strength training to elite athletes and power lifters who employ this to enhance sport-specific strength. This type of exercise is highly dangerous for everybody else! It is critical that you use the correct technique and form in performing any strength exercises. Again, the guidance of an experienced, qualified trainer will not only protect you from injury, but also ensure that you get maximal benefit from each exercise.

Perhaps the most important muscle groups for you to strengthen are those that support your core. Your abdominal and back muscles provide vital strength and stabilization for your spine, which is not only the basis of all movement but also protects your spinal cord and the important nerves that supply sensation and motion to the rest of your body. Fortunately, abdominal and back exercises have received a lot of popular attention recently, and whether you participate in a thirty-day plank challenge or enjoy exercising while balanced on top of a giant fitness ball, there are a lot of fun ways to achieve this important fitness objective.

THE POWER OF FLEXIBILITY: COMBATTING AGING

One of the features of age- and inactivity-related decay is a loss of joint mobility, or stiffness. It has both a physical and a psychological impact on your WHealth. Interestingly, unlike aerobic and strength training that have largely physical benefits plus bonus mental and emotional benefits, flexibility may be most valuable for non-physical reasons. I realize that this is a subjective position, and very hard to substantiate with research, but there is little doubt in my mind that declining flexibility is a significant opponent to a youthful disposition. If you groan when you get out of bed in the morning, or struggle to look over your shoulder while you reverse your car, or can no longer cut your toenails, you begin to feel old. When you feel old, you believe that you're getting old. You want to avoid feelings of aging at all costs. My strong recommendation is that you include flexibility training in your life to combat these feelings of aging.

The goal of flexibility training is to increase and maintain a good range of motion in the major joints and their surrounding muscle-tendon groups. Research shows that this goal can be achieved at all ages. Flexibility increases temporarily after a single bout of stretching and improves in an enduring fashion after three to four weeks of regular stretching. In addition to the psychological benefits (when you feel young, you act young) and practical benefits (you can tie your shoelaces again), research has demonstrated several physical benefits. In particular, stretching enhances stability and balance in your posture. Flexibility training helps special nerves (called *proprioceptive nerves*) keep joints in the right position, which is critical for their stability and control.

I recommend that you include flexibility training in your regimen two to three times per week. You can develop a good routine that only takes you ten minutes, which will likely fit easily into your schedule. Plus, it's good for your body and your mind!

As with resistance training, there are many ways to perform flexibility training. Currently, there is a surge in the popularity of yoga, tai chi, and a host of similar low-impact exercise forms that involve a combination of relaxation, resistance, and flexibility training, often with significant mental, emotional, and spiritual exercise. I'm a big fan of all these disciplines! Unless you're involved in fast-moving sessions that are more aerobically challenging, you can't really use them as substantial components of your 10,000 steps, but their emotional, flexibility, and strength benefits are considerable and well worth your time.

Although stretching is a lower-risk form of exercise than strength training, I generally still recommend that you start your flexibility training with a good trainer. Often, the same expert who guides you in your resistance training can help with your flexibility prescription. The reason that I advocate for this is that there are many ways to achieve flexibility, and not all are good. You have to find the right type of exercises, ranges of motion, and durations of stretches for your individual condition and requirements. There are many good online resources that can help you, so don't let the lack of access to a fancy trainer keep you from stretching. As always, my advice if you're starting up after a long break, or have underlying physical limitations, is to seek medical advice first!

KEY #2: COUNT CALORIES

Count calories to balance your energy.

I could tell you a lot of scary things about being overweight. I could tell you that over 20 percent of heart attacks and over 60 percent of diabetes cases are attributable to being overweight. I could tell you that *adipocytes* (fat cells) play a sinister role in systemic inflammation that drives high blood pressure and stroke. I could tell you that excessive weight increases your risk of developing cancer of the colon, breast, uterus, and gallbladder. I could tell you that it increases the chance of your experiencing osteoarthritis.

But I won't, because you probably are already acutely conscious of this, and spend time worrying about it, and bounce between various programs trying to lose weight. I know, because I did. And worse than all of this, I bet you feel bad despite your efforts! Most of us just feel unhappy when we can't fit into our clothes or the mirror shows us things we don't want to see. As a physician, I knew all the scary facts, but I only took meaningful, lasting action after sitting in exquisite pain for six interminable hours, stuffed into a tiny seat on a transcontinental flight, feeling like I couldn't breathe. I felt trapped, both physically and emotionally. It was time to make big changes!

Few people will argue that being a healthy weight is a good second step (after exercise) for achieving BodyWHealth. But how do you get there?

You achieve your healthy weight by mastering the simple, yet delicate, energy balance that governs the life of every single organism, including humans. Now, when I talk about energy, I'm not talking about the dynamic feeling you have when you're not fatigued (although there is a relationship between how you feel and what you eat). What I'm talking about is fuel for your body, which scientists call "energy." It's the currency for living. To breathe, eat, work, or play, we burn energy. In turn, we must replenish our energy stores by eating.

Scientists study something called "energetics" at top universities and labs. One profoundly simple equation rules all of their work: The amount of energy you take in *must* balance the amount of energy you use. If it doesn't, then your weight changes. It's very, very simple. No matter what fancy diet you choose to follow, this is the *only* important rule for weight control! If you take in more energy than you're using for a sustained period of time, you will store the excess as fat and compromise your BodyWHealth.

THE ROOT OF THE PROBLEM

For a long time, scientists considered fat cells to be just that: cells full of fat. We believed that all they did was store fat. We knew that metabolic energy from many sources was converted into fat, a convenient storage form. Those fat molecules were then carefully packaged in specialized cells called adipocytes. A bit like the warehouses that manage inventory for Amazon, these adipocytes were situated around the body at convenient places, especially under the skin and around our internal organs. When we needed energy and didn't have energy-rich sugar readily available, or preferred a more efficient energy source (fat requires less oxygen than sugar to burn for energy), our body called on those fat stores to release some of their precious reserves for our immediate use.

This is a beautiful system, and it worked extremely well when we were hunter-gatherers roaming the plains. When we caught a big meal, we feasted and packed the excess energy into our portable energy stores (adipocytes) for later use when food wasn't as plentiful. The system worked because life was very different then. First, we exercised a lot—all the time, actually. After sleeping off our big meal, we knew we had to get going, and we did. There was work to be done: hard physical work. This meant we used those fat stores up quickly, before they had the chance to make us overweight. Second, for the most part, food was neither as plentiful nor as convenient as it is for modern humans. This meant we weren't eating enough of those big meals to make us overweight.

But then our lifestyle changed and rapidly outstripped the pace of our biological evolution. We in developed countries soon found ourselves living in calorie excess, surrounded by convenient, refined foods produced in bulk for the masses. It was the modern era that heralded room service, convenience stores, and fast food, where a few dollars could buy a massive 900-calorie, high-fat snack. And on top of that, we were no longer exercising! By using simple math, you can figure out that we started consuming more energy than we were burning, and our fat cells kept doing the job they were designed to do: packing away the excess energy until they were bulging at their seams and we were bulging out of our clothes.

Scientists noticed that people who weighed more and who had more fat than others lived shorter lives and were affected more often by cardiovascular and metabolic diseases. We noticed that they had more heart attacks, had higher blood pressure, and developed type 2 diabetes at a younger age. It was not difficult to understand how a bigger body would require the heart and blood vessels to work harder, but we couldn't explain the emergence of diabetes.

So we went back into the labs and the clinics to find better answers. There is a lot we still need to learn, but increasingly, it appears that these little adipocytes really aren't as inert as we thought. They do more than provide fat storage. We now know them to be complex metabolic units that react very badly to the abuse they suffer as a result of our modern lifestyle.

It turns out that fat cells are intimately linked to the inflammatory crisis created by our high-calorie, low-exercise lifestyle. When we eat a high-calorie meal, especially if it is also high in saturated fat, we can measure a surge of pro-inflammatory agents in our blood. In fact, high blood sugar alone is enough to trigger the release of the most famous of all pro-inflammatory fiends: IL6. (You will hopefully remember IL6 to be the leader of the destructive forces that drive degeneration and decay.) While these IL6 surges are short-lived (and probably happened when our ancestors feasted, too), a real problem arises when the frequency of calorie overload increases. With a modern diet and repetitive overeating, these short-lived surges follow one another in rapid succession, inducing an enduring elevation in IL6 and other pro-inflammatory cytokines.

It would be bad enough if that were the full story. Sadly, there is more to it: Something happens at the level of the adipocytes themselves that exacerbates the inflammation significantly. The bloated fat cells appear to let out a desperate cry for help. It's almost as though they turn to our immune systems asking for help. And by now, I bet you can guess how the immune system responds. You're right—with inflammation!

We know from studying fat cells that they become factories of pro-inflammatory cytokines when overloaded by a high-calorie diet. They send out distress signals, and the immune system reacts as though the body is in danger. It activates inflammatory cells, the agents of degeneration and decay, and sends them streaming around the body to perform their destructive duties.

And that's not all! The curious part of this story is that another chemical, called *leptin*, gets involved. Leptin is a signaling protein more popularly known as the "satiety hormone." When we eat, leptin levels rise, eventually telling our brains that we've had enough. The natural response is to stop eating. But we live in unnatural circumstances today, where we force-feed ourselves beyond natural boundaries. We continue to eat, despite rising leptin levels. In response, our overloaded adipocytes pump out even more leptin, desperately trying to get us to stop. It appears that this excess leptin plays a central role in eliciting "help" from the immune system. Bulging fat cells secrete leptin in an almost desperate attempt to get us to stop eating, and when we don't listen, they call in the demolition gangs. You will remember that these pro-inflammatory cytokines are dedicated and enthusiastic workers that only stop when the anti-inflammatory cytokines show up. The good news is that exercise stimulates the production of those anti-inflammatory forces that are the only natural means of controlling the activity of the pro-inflammatory army. The problem is that we tend to calorie-overload in the absence of exercise. Our bodies activate the army of decay without simultaneously activating the army of regeneration. The imbalance in forces has disastrous consequences.

So, can we now explain the link between inflammation of fat cells and diabetes? Not completely, although our insight is advancing rapidly. It appears that the engorged and irritated fat cells stop taking in excess fat, and may even become a little leaky, either because they have simply had enough and overflow, or because inflammation affects the integrity of the adipocyte walls that usually keep the fat inside the cells. Either way, the overflow fat is sucked in at other sites by other cells, such as liver and skeletal muscle cells, where it interferes with those cells' sensitivity to insulin, the chief regulator of sugar metabolism. We call this "insulin resistance." It triggers a cascade of nasty metabolic consequences, and you start to slide down the slippery slope of metabolic syndrome, pre-diabetes, and ultimately full-blown type 2 diabetes!

There is some intriguing science about leptin that seems eerily similar to the story of insulin resistance in diabetes. It appears that under conditions of systemic inflammatory overload, your body may become resistant to leptin the same way it can become resistant to insulin. This means that your brain

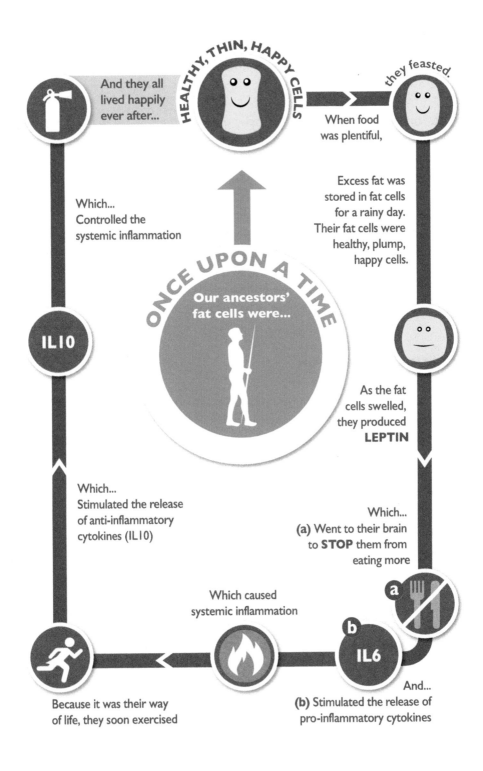

no longer responds to the stop-eating signal sent from the bulging fat cells. We need more research to fully understand this phenomenon, and whether it is largely a cause or effect of the metabolic syndrome. Regardless, it's a pretty scary thought.

With fat stores now becoming factories of inflammation, circulating levels of pro-inflammatory cytokines rise two to three times higher than the healthy natural levels. Visceral (or abdominal) fat is the biggest problem. Large amounts of belly fat, measured via abdominal girth, is highly correlated with the ugly consequences of systemic inflammation, especially cardiovascular disease, type 2 diabetes, colon cancer, and breast cancer—even in people with normal body weight! Let me repeat this last nuance in case you missed it, because most people believe that only extreme obesity exposes you to health risk. Not true! Recent research[9] has shown that an increase in belly fat is associated with an increase in disease risk, regardless of actual weight. Belly fat, *regardless of body weight*, is highly dangerous!

PORTION DISTORTION

That's enough science for now. But there is one more problem we need to explore before we can discuss solutions: portion size. We're not only sedentary and eating refined foods loaded with too many saturated fats and calories, but we're also simply eating too much!

"I can't eat the way I could twenty years ago!" Have you heard people say this? I have. Most times, the person saying it will blame the aging process. While it's true that your metabolic rate slows a little as you age, there is another shocking truth that explains this sad phenomenon: changes in portion size.

Portion sizes have grown dramatically over the past twenty years. In some cases, they have tripled! So if you happily ate a modest turkey sandwich each day for lunch at the corner deli twenty years ago, without putting on weight, know that the calorie load of your lunch has probably more than doubled since then. It has probably increased 2.6 times, to be precise. Data[10,11] shared by the National Institutes of Health (NIH) and the National Heart, Lung, and Blood Institute (NHLBI) in the USA and the British Heart Foundation in the UK expose this horrendous trend. The data in the table below show the calorie content of some common foods twenty years ago and the massively inflated calorie content of the same foods today. Both portion size and calorie density have increased.

TODAY
Living a modern lifestyle,
our fat cells are...

Tired, bloated and overworked.
Food is always plentiful,
and we indulge, often...

Stuffing more and more fat
into our strained adipocytes...

 LEPTIN LEPTIN LEPTIN

That desperately pump out
Leptin as fast as they can

BUT... Our brain is no longer
sensitive to Leptin's persistent
pleas to have us stop eating

AND... Because we no longer exercise

The flood of pro-inflammatory
cytokines (IL6) is now unopposed

 Causing Systemic Inflammatory OVERLOAD

Which results in
DEGENERATION
and DECAY

**Our overloaded fat cells leak fat
into muscle and liver cells, causing
insulin insensitivity and diabetes**

CALORIE INFLATION OVER 20 YEARS

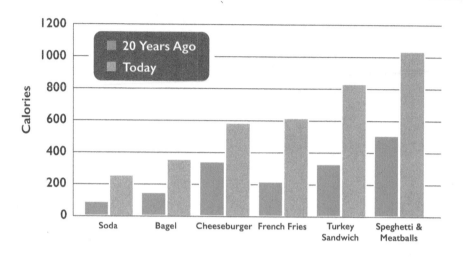

To offset this calorie inflation, we clearly need to be more disciplined about exercise habits. We have to exercise even more than our ancestors did to burn the additional calories of portion overload. The infographic below estimates the additional exercise required to burn off the excess calories associated with today's portion distortion. Perhaps retro-menus will become fashionable one day, but until then, it is far more sensible for WHealth Seekers to *both* reduce their potion size *and* increase exercise. As you know by now, these actions have complementary benefits in quelling the inflammatory fire that has become the modern Achilles' heel.

THE DIET DOWNFALL

So now that you've heard about the dangers of being overweight and falling victim to portion distortion, you're probably ready to jump headfirst into a diet, right? If so, you're not alone. The customary response to feeling overweight is to dive into a "diet." The problem is that, for the vast majority of people, these short-term calorie purges don't work—and there are three main reasons why.

The first reason is that your metabolism slows down to prevent weight loss. The body requires *glucose* (sugar) for energy. Under normal circumstances, we take glucose that is circulating in our blood and move it into our cells to fuel our metabolic needs. When we have inadequate glucose in the blood, we

SUBSTANTIAL ADDITIONAL EXERCISE IS REQUIRED TO OFFSET THE CALORIE EXCESS DUE TO PORTION INFLATION

1990	TODAY	Extra Exercise Required	
		WALK (mins)	RUN (mins)
BAGEL x 2.5		32	21
TURKEY SANDWICH x 2.6		75	50
BURGER x 1.8		39	26
FRIES x 2.9		60	40
SPAGHETTI x 2.1		79	53
SODA x 2.9		25	17

mobilize it from the liver and muscle tissue, where it is stockpiled in a special storage form known as *glycogen*. Once the glycogen stores are depleted, the body is forced to break down first fat (from adipocytes) and then protein (from muscles) to produce glucose to meet its energy needs. This is the theory behind a diet where you achieve a sustained negative calorie balance—you force your body to raid your fat reserves for energy.

As a result of this knowledge, people starve themselves in the hopes of burning off their fat. But the body is smart. When it detects a substantial reduction in calorie intake, it adapts to protect itself. Your brain may know that you will eventually feed your body again, but your body doesn't. Your body thinks that the calorie restriction may last forever, and in fear of starvation, it activates a primal defense mechanism and slows down your metabolism. Now you go from a bad situation to a worse situation: Your body is now resisting your valiant efforts to lose weight!

Compare this to the impact of exercise on your body. Your metabolic rate increases both during and after exercise. Increased metabolic rate means more calories burned, even at rest. With exercise, you get your body working *with* you to lose weight!

The second reason that diets don't work is that with a low-volume diet, you always feel hungry. Most low-calorie diets are also low-volume diets, which require you to eat less. The stomach has stretch receptors that send messages via nerves to the brain when you have eaten enough to sustain life. These messages induce chemical changes in the *satiety* center in your brain, and your body knows it should stop eating.

When you go on a low-volume diet, you no longer trigger the stretch receptors in your stomach, and so you always feel hungry. That's an unhappy, counter-productive state. You now associate "healthy behavior" with misery. That's neither a reward nor an incentive. Actually, it's a big turn-off! It's better for you to eat bulky foods that are relatively low in calories. Plant-based, fiber-rich diets are high in volume and low in calories. You would need to eat a whole pound of fruits, vegetables, and whole grains to ingest even 500 to 600 calories. While eating fiber-rich foods still restricts calories (but not drastically enough to invoke the starvation response), it also triggers your stretch receptors, so you don't feel hungry all the time. You now *associate healthy eating with healthy emotion.* Unlike a low-volume diet, this is sustainable.

The final reason diets fail is that most of them are driven by negative emotions. The most dangerous thing about a crash diet is the deep emotional sabotage you invoke. You need to be highly motivated to adhere to a diet like this. Few people get this motivation from an overwhelming desire for a healthy, slim body. The vast majority motivate themselves using deep *hatred* for their current body. In this hatred, they embark on a vengeful journey, punishing their body with denial and starvation. Worse still, failure to lose weight is met with a surge in hatred. You're angry with yourself for failing, and you assume that you didn't hate yourself enough in the first place. So you fill your head with more deeply hurtful, undermining self-judgment. In an avalanche of self-hatred, your one-cookie mistake becomes a seven-cookie feast, and you lie on the couch in a stew of self-pity and misery, hoping to feel good enough about yourself to start over again in the morning. And so on. And if you do hate yourself successfully and stick to your draconian diet for long enough to lose weight, guess what happens next? You rebound emotionally.

Having achieved your goal, you stop hating, and in celebration you resume the original eating habits that got you in trouble in the first place.

Contrast this with the body's own design for behavior modification: *serotonin*. Serotonin is the "feel-good" hormone in our bodies. It's a powerful chemical reward system that drives feelings of happiness and contentment. When the brain releases serotonin, in response to exercise for example, you feel great! You begin to desire this feeling and will do whatever you need to release more serotonin. So, you exercise more. This is positive reinforcement. It's how your body is built. If *you* treat your body with the same affirmation, it will reward you.

By now you can see how I'm hoping we as WHealth Seekers will approach attaining a healthy weight: In order to achieve a sustainable healthy weight, you must implement enduring, balanced lifestyle modifications. If you need to lose weight to achieve BodyWHealth, be kind to your body. Picture and admire it in its future state. *Believe!* You're going to hear a lot more about belief in the next section of this book. Use powerful positive thinking, together with inspiring emotional visualization, and you will achieve sustainable healthy changes. Improve your calorie balance by first burning more fuel. Exercise! If that is not enough, then *slowly* nudge your metabolism into negative balance. Gradually reduce your food intake until you have a negative daily balance that you can sustain for long enough to reach your goal. This subtle shift prevents the body from going into a counter-productive starvation mode. Eat nutritious, high-fiber foods that keep the stretch receptors in your stomach firing, so you don't feel hungry. And then, when you reach your goal, gradually shift back toward a neutral balance where you eat what you burn, and no more, and no less.

YOUR PRESCRIPTION FOR WHEALTH

Now that you've heard the sobering message about fat and diet, I'd like to share a few pieces of very exciting news with you.

First, research has shown that significant reductions in pro-inflammatory cytokines and significant increases in anti-inflammatory cytokines are present within four weeks of starting a very-low-calorie diet.[12] Please note that I'm not suggesting a very-low-calorie diet. As I mentioned above, I'm a fan of a more modest, gradual approach—getting your body to work with you and not against you. But the fantastic truth is that you can tip your inflammatory balance back in favor of rejuvenation and youth by modifying your diet!

More important, from my perspective, is the second piece of news: that you are able to reverse the risk of inflammatory disease regardless of your starting weight.[13] This is excellent news if you are significantly overweight, and it is very good news if you are close to your target weight but still have a little belly fat. You should have been alarmed when you read earlier that your risk of disease is elevated when you have excess visceral fat, regardless of your actual weight. The fact that we can *all* reverse this risk is one of the more exciting BodyWHealth facts!

The final piece of good news is that energy is a simple balance. You consume energy in the form of calories from your diet and burn it in your daily activities. When you consume more than you burn, you store the excess as fat. When you burn more than you consume, you need to retrieve energy (in the form of fat) from your fat stores to make up the difference. I repeat, when you burn more energy than you consume, you have to remove fat from your fat stores. That's the magic!

So, how do we achieve this energy balance that will restore us to good health regardless of our starting points? Simply by following BodyWHealth's second Key: *Count calories to balance your energy.* In addition to taking 10,000 steps on at least five days of each week for the rest of your life, I believe that this is the most valuable thing you can do to achieve the appropriate energy balance and control your weight. In doing so, you will eliminate surplus energy intake and reduce any excess weight you carry, especially in the form of belly fat—a huge win for all WHealth Seekers!

You might be wondering why I would choose to focus on calories. Why don't I just tell you to lose weight? It's because tracking the calories you consume and burn has been shown in high-quality scientific studies[14] to make a meaningful difference in your diet, and more importantly in your weight. If you have a desire to control your weight and you make the effort to track your calorie intake, your chances of being successful in losing weight increase between 30 and 50 percent!

The reason is simple; it's all about awareness. One of the biggest dangers of food consumption today is that we eat in an automated fashion, grabbing whatever is there, whatever is most convenient, whatever everybody else is eating. In contrast, when you track what you eat, you are highly conscious of your meal size, content, and frequency. You're a smart person, and you make smart decisions. You now eat *mindfully*. You can almost double your success in controlling your energy balance by simply counting your calories.

So, *how* do you estimate your calorie intake and energy output to make sure you're achieving the perfect balance? The first step is to keep an accurate log of everything you eat and all of your exercise. Particularly if you are a novice at counting calories, it is vital that you write everything down! Now, this probably won't sound particularly appealing as you sit down to eat the lovely dinner Grandma just made—especially since she probably didn't put a nutrition label with calorie counts on the plate! You'll probably just want to enjoy your meal, and you should. But once you're done, write down what you've eaten, even if you don't feel like it. Use a napkin, a spreadsheet, an app, or a program, but capture this information! Do the same every time you exercise. You'll wind up with an excellent record that will enable you to move to the next step in calculating your energy balance.

The next step is to add up your total intake and output at the end of each day. That way, you'll know how much energy you are consuming and burning each day, and you can evaluate your energy balance. You can see on a daily basis if you are eating more energy than you burn, or burning more than you eat. If your intake exceeds your burn rate, I guarantee you will end up overweight. If your intake is less than your burn rate, I guarantee you will lose weight. Period!

Now, you're probably wondering exactly how you can determine those intake and output figures. Let's start with estimating how much energy you are *taking in* each day: that is, how many calories are in the food you eat. When I started my own quest for BodyWHealth in earnest, I downloaded seven calorie-calculator apps onto my mobile phone and signed up for another five online services. In my enthusiasm, I wanted to find the one that worked best for me. I found two apps to be the most useful: The first logged my calorie intake and my exercise and helped me balance my energy load; the second scanned the bar code on food packaging and gave me information about its calorie content, as well as rating the quality of the food. You will find a large number of other tools available. Choose the one that works for you. (If you'd like to know which apps I'm currently using, please visit my blog.) There are also countless books and online references that list the number of calories in commonly eaten foods. And don't forget about the nutrition labels on packaged foods—those are incredibly useful tools that you should always read! It really doesn't matter which resources you use as long as you are estimating your calorie intake.

Now let's talk about how to estimate how much energy you are *burning* each day. Energy consumption takes place in three different processes. The first is the basic energy we need to simply keep us alive, known as *Basal Metabolic Rate (BMR)*. Our organs and tissues are constantly active, even while we sleep. This metabolic activity consumes energy regardless of our physical activity levels. For most of us, it accounts for the bulk of the energy we consume in any one day. BMR is largely dependent on our size and age, although there is some variability between similar individuals. Our BMR starts extremely high when we are rapidly growing and developing babies, and stays relatively high into early adulthood. It then declines gradually throughout the rest of our lives (with a decrease of about 20 percent from the age of twenty to the age of seventy). This accounts for our tendency to put on weight more easily as we grow older.

The second process is the *energy consumption of activity*. This is the additional energy we burn to fuel our exercise. It is voluntary energy expenditure and goes up or down depending on our daily activities. Finally, in the third process, we expend a tiny amount of additional energy in digesting our food, known as the *thermic effect of food*. We count this separately from our BMR because it varies depending on the nature and size of each meal. If we don't eat, then there is no energy required for digestion. On the other hand, a huge meal with coarse grains or tough meat requires more energy for digestion.

There are many good BMR calculators[15] available online that will estimate your BMR based on your height, weight, age, and gender. The same calculators then use a conversion to estimate your total energy consumption by including what you've burned using the other two processes. You can use an average daily estimate as your daily burn rate, or you can estimate the energy you burn each day (which is more accurate because a day of rest will differ from a 10,000-step day). Either way, you need this estimate because it will help you determine how much energy you are taking in versus how much you are expending.

BALANCED CALORIE EQUATION

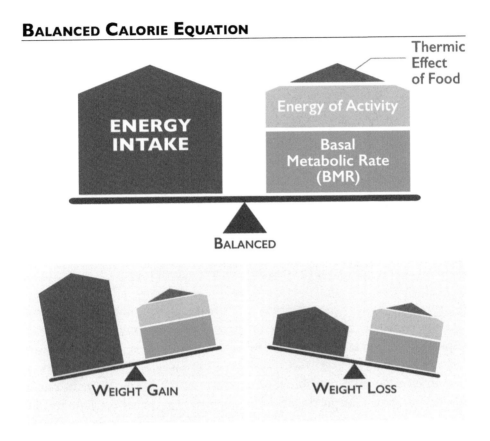

OVERCOMING THE CALORIE-COUNTING IMPERFECTIONS

You'll notice that I frequently use the word "estimate" when I refer to the science of calorie counting. That's because your calorie calculations will only ever be estimates at best. Critics of the process will tell you not to waste your time counting calories, because you won't be accurate anyway. I agree that you won't be perfectly accurate (and I'll explain why in a minute); I don't agree, however, that that makes it a waste of time.

The best way scientists have to measure the calorie content of food is to burn it in a special chamber (called a *calorimeter*) that measures the heat energy emitted during its combustion. When we do this, we get accurate measures of the calorie load in that food. Unfortunately, this doesn't give us a good estimate of the calories that your body actually gets from eating that food. Some foods are harder to break down, like nuts or meat, and we don't fully extract all the calories during regular digestion. A calorimeter would overestimate the calories you take in by eating these hard-to-digest foods. You would also use more energy to digest these tough foods than you might in digesting other foods. The calorimeter would not measure this extra energy burn, so the final measure would be a double overestimate of the effective calorie load you take in by eating a handful of nuts, for example.

To make it more complicated, digestion varies between individuals, so even if we were able to estimate the energy an average person gets from a specific food, it wouldn't necessarily be accurate for *you*. The bacterial content of your gut plays a significant role in digestion, and this content varies considerably between individuals, and even over time in the same individual. Cooking and processing of foods also alter the amount of calories present and the proportion of them that are available to us, so even the scientific gold standard is only going to provide you with a rough estimate.

Another, more worrying, barrier to fully accurate calorie counting is that the reported calorie content of many foods you buy—whether at a restaurant, from a fast-food chain, or in the grocery store—are inaccurate. The Department of Agriculture oversees compliance with the nutrition facts in commercially available food products in the USA. They tolerate a 20-percent error in reporting. So, the nutrition fact panel on your box of cereal can be either over- or underreporting the cereal's calorie load by as much as 20 percent, and still be legal. An alarming study[16] published in the *Journal of the American Dietetic Association* found that, on average, restaurants underestimate the calorie content of food by 18 percent. The study only evaluated "low-calorie" meals, so this may be the tip of a sizeable iceberg. Not only are portion sizes growing, but the official estimates of calorie content are overlooking almost 100 calories for every 500-calorie meal.

Despite all these hindrances to perfectly accurate calculations, I stick to my calorie-counting recommendation passionately. The second Key to WHealth is not about scientific precision. It's about mindfulness. Remember, you double the chance of success in controlling your weight by simply counting your calories, whether you have a completely accurate total or not. There are few other interventions known to modern science that will give you this much bang for your buck. So please, count calories!

COUNTING CALORIES TO A LOWER WEIGHT

When people need to lose weight, scientists advocate for a negative calorie balance of between 500 and 1,000 calories per day. This means that their energy consumption must be higher than their intake by between 500 and 1,000 calories per day. They could achieve the 500-calorie target by reducing their intake by 250 calories per day (that's a candy bar or a small serving of fries) *and* increasing their exercise consumption by 250 calories per day (that's a thirty-minute bike ride or a forty-five-minute moderate-paced

EQUATION FOR ESTIMATING DAILY CALORIC (ENERGY) BALANCE

ENERGY INTAKE:	ENERGY CONSUMPTION:
# Calories in breakfast	# Calories burned in regular daily activities (BMR)
+ # Calories in lunch	+ # Calories burned to digest food *
+ # Calories in dinner	+ # Calories burned during exercise
+ # Calories in snacks	
+ # Calories in beverages	
= TOTAL ENERGY INTAKE (in calories)	= TOTAL ENERGY CONSUMPTION (in calories)

ENERGY (CALORIC) BALANCE

When your ...

Intake	Intake	Intake
- Consumption	- Consumption	- Consumption
= Positive	= Zero	= Negative

Then you ...

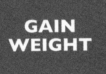 GAIN WEIGHT	MAINTAIN WEIGHT	LOSE WEIGHT

* For our purposes, there is no need to estimate the energy required to digest your food. So, Consumption = BMR + Exercise

walk). They will lose 3,500 calories per week, which is roughly equivalent to one pound of fat per week.

I do have a strong word of caution about losing weight, however: Not everybody's body responds to calorie restriction and increased exercise in the same way. There can be considerable variability between individuals in their response to calorie restriction and exercise. So, you and your friend who weigh the same, eat the same, and exercise the same may end up losing weight at different rates.

The reason for this is that there are two different metabolic responses to calorie restriction[17]: a "thrifty phenotype," in which the body reduces its BMR to protect itself against energy deficiency, and a "spendthrift" metabolism that loses weight more rapidly. In those with thrifty phenotypes, the body sometimes compensates for the reduction in energy intake and/or the increase in energy consumption, trying to protect itself by conserving energy, either by modifying appetite or BMR, or both. This can be a frustrating problem for those WHealth Seekers intent on losing weight who don't see results as rapidly as they'd like.

RESPONSES TO CALORIE RESTRICTION

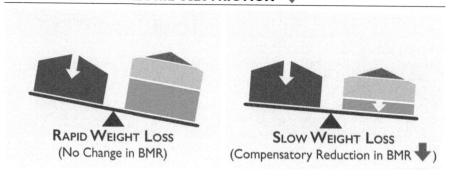

RAPID WEIGHT LOSS
(No Change in BMR)

SLOW WEIGHT LOSS
(Compensatory Reduction in BMR)

Similarly, there are two different metabolic responses to the increased energy demand of exercise.[18] In some cases, the body reduces its BMR to protect itself against an increase in the energy demand of exercise. Again, this can be frustrating. The important thing is not to get discouraged. Remember that you are on your journey to WHealth, and that you will get there!

RESPONSES TO INCREASE IN EXERCISE

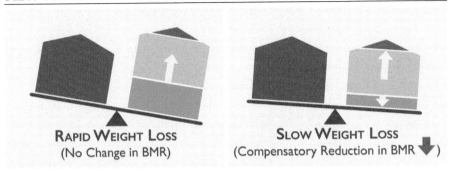

RAPID WEIGHT LOSS
(No Change in BMR)

SLOW WEIGHT LOSS
(Compensatory Reduction in BMR ⬇)

FREEING YOURSELF FROM THE SCALE

I have one final note of warning before you embark on your calorie-counting journey. You may be surprised that I didn't advocate that your most important gadget (after your step counter) be your bathroom scale. This is very deliberate. I won't often tell you to lose weight, but I will often urge you toward BodyWHealth. There is a subtle but immensely powerful difference.

I realize that this advice may be controversial, and may seem counter-intuitive to you, but I feel very strongly about this: *Get rid of your bathroom scale!* It is more dangerous to you than it is worth.

Not only has the same science that proved the value of counting calories shown that self-weighing is far less helpful, but it has also shown that self-weighing can actually be very dangerous. There are several reasons for this.

First, self-weighing diverts your focus to the wrong end of the problem. Your weight is not the problem; what you're eating is. Focus your attention on your plate, not the scale!

Each time you focus on your weight, you reinforce the problem and the pain. Later in this book, you will learn about the power of belief. If you look at the scale and it tells you you're overweight, you'll believe it. In fact, each time you see that number, you'll believe it more. What you believe becomes true, and you'll become locked in a seemingly inescapable, exceedingly painful prison. It makes you feel guilty and sad, and then your discipline and resolve is eroded and you make poor eating decisions. This reverberating cycle of gloom is hard to escape.

With a scale, you focus on a number, not a destination. Your destination is to look good and feel good. Keep that image in your mind.

The habit of standing on the scale triggers old mindsets and habits. After reading this book, you will be inspired to live differently. Getting back onto the scale will suck you back into the unhealthy past.

Your weight is a fluctuating number, and a poor predictor of health anyway. Your amount of fluid intake and the timing of your last meal or bowel movement influence your weight at any one moment, with no change in your actual body fat. This can trick and depress you, making weight a relatively poor measure of your WHealth.

More important to your WHealth than your weight is your body fat percentage, especially your amount of belly fat. Your bathroom mirror and the fit of your clothes will tell you far more about this than your bathroom scale.

Finally, you want to be in control of your destiny. You have an excellent view of what you desire, and you're the best person to be driving yourself toward that goal. When you enslave yourself to your bathroom scale, you give *it* the power. Don't do it.

I suggest that you weigh yourself very occasionally in your doctor's office or a pharmacy that has a good-quality scale. You need a vague sense of where you're at and what your target is. But that's all. The healthiest way is for you to find a happy path to weight loss, and the bathroom scale, even if hidden by your bathrobe hanging in the corner, is not your friend!

SIMPLE RECOMMENDATIONS FOR COUNTING CALORIES

1. *Listen to your body.* Each of us is different, and our metabolisms may respond differently to the same calorie balance. You own body may even have fluctuations over time in the way it handles specific food or exercise loads. Your best guide is your own experience. Close awareness of your calorie balance and your body's response to it will help you to manage your weight appropriately.

2. *Use both diet and exercise.* If you want to lose weight, increase your exercise *and* reduce your calorie intake. If, for example, you reduce your calorie intake by 500 calories per day without doing any additional exercise, you may be more likely to induce a protective response from your body.

3. *Start slow.* You probably don't want to hear this, but it may take longer than you had hoped to reach your goal weight. You must prevent your body from slipping into energy-conservation mode. Aim for a negative balance of only 250 calories per day, and see how it works. It may be that less-extreme energy deprivation results in a less rigorous compensatory response, and you'll actually lose weight faster.

4. *Focus on feeling.* Don't focus on your weight, but rather on how you feel. In case you didn't catch this already, I don't like the bathroom scale! You should have a vague idea of your actual weight and your goal weight, but don't obsess over them. It is far more important how you feel about yourself. Most of us care more about how we look and feel and how our clothes fit us than the number on the scale, anyway.

5. *Be patient.* It's fantastic that you *are* losing weight and taking steps on your BodyWHealth journey, even if you're progressing slower than you'd like. Check your equations, and make sure that your calculations are correct. Then hunker down for the long haul. You're doing great things for your health, even if your weight is taking a while to respond. And when you reach your goal, you're far more likely to maintain it, in part because of the fantastic diligence that has gotten you there!

CONCLUSION

At first, calorie counting is a difficult task, and it might be a challenge to put in the initial hard work to derive the long-term reward. In the end, I can assure you from personal experience that the job becomes quick and easy. Today, I look at a plate and can guess with sufficient accuracy its calorie content. I know what my basic BMR is, and I know how much energy an hour of walking, running, kayaking, or swimming burns. Without the labor of writing or calculating, I can tell each day if I'm over or under on my balance. In the end, that's all you need. And if you ever get despondent, remember that the taste of BodyWHealth is highly addicting! It is worth every bit of this hard work. Once you've tasted it, you'll never want to let it go.

You are now an expert in two of the three Keys to physical WHealth. I hope that you are practicing what you're learning!

In addition to counting the calories you take in each day, I advocate that you address two common challenges to healthy, calorie-balanced eating habits: drinking high-calorie beverages and eating emotionally.

THE POWER OF DRINKING WELL: AN EASY WAY TO CUT CALORIES

One of the places calories creep into our diets is in our drinks. Over the last three decades, America's calorie intake from sweetened drinks has increased over 30 percent. The average person consumes around 200 calories per day from sodas, sweetened teas and coffee, fruit drinks, sport drinks, and "low-calorie" beverages. Add 100 calories per day from alcohol, and you get to an average consumption per adult of 300 calories per day. That's more than 10 percent of the generally recommended daily allowance of around 2,000 calories. If we can control the intake of these sweetened drinks, that's a big step toward maintaining a healthy daily energy balance.

Many nutrition scientists talk about "empty calories." This refers to the ingestion of calories from a food or beverage that provides little additional nutritional value. If you eat a juicy steak, for example, it is loaded with calories, but at least you're getting some necessary protein, too. If you drink a soda, on the other hand, all you're getting are calories, with no additional nutritional value. Most calorie-loaded drinks are full of these empty calories—even the ones marketed as being "healthy."

There are several ways to limit your consumption of these empty, calorie-loaded beverages. *First, you can track your liquid calorie intake.* If you're not actively tracking your liquid intake (and until you are experienced in this, I mean recording it in a calorie diary), you will not be mindful of it, and excess calories can easily creep into your diet.

Take note of the number of calories you're consuming every week from sweetened drinks. If you want a graphic, eye-opening shock, then add up the number of extra sugar calories you're drinking and convert it into the table sugar equivalent (one teaspoon is 15 calories). Then measure out the equivalent quantity of sugar into a breakfast bowl to visualize the excess. You will be amazed. Your average daily consumption of 300 calories is equivalent to twenty teaspoons of sugar!

Reduce your sweetened drink intake. You'd be astonished at the number of drinks that contain extra sugar. If you drink a couple of cups of coffee every day, with a couple of teaspoons of sugar in each, you soon consume an extra 60 to 80 calories. You'd have to exercise for ten to fifteen minutes per day just to work this excess off! Soda is also brimming with sugar. Walking off a single soda will take you twenty to thirty minutes. You should be particularly wary of sports drinks. I see kids drinking them for refreshment because their parents see them as "healthy." But in fact, they are loaded with sugar—good for heavy exercise, but bad for BodyWHealth. Another sugar- and calorie-loaded beverage masquerading as healthy, whole milk contains double the calories of nonfat milk, and much more sugar (natural sugar is still sugar). Finally, alcohol is also loaded with sugar and calories. A single beer will require twenty-five minutes to walk off. A glass of red wine every day is good for you (even recommended), but remember that it contains about 125 calories, so you will have to make space for it somewhere else in your diet. Hard liquor has the highest calorie concentration at about 100 calories per single shot.

Drink water! Start the day with a glass and end the day with a glass. Drink a glass before every meal. Often, we eat because we're thirsty, so this will help to avoid the other empty calories that tempt you. If you drink water before a meal, it also distends your stomach a little so that the stretch receptors are triggered earlier, and you'll eat less.

Finally, be wary of artificial sweeteners. Many physicians are supportive of sweeteners that replace raw sugar in drinks. However, recent evidence suggests that they may also be associated with a higher prevalence of diabetes, hinting that they affect the pancreas and insulin metabolism in a manner similar to raw sugar. My strong preference is that WHealth Seekers wean themselves off any dependence on sweet taste.

As long as you balance your calories, you can include some sweetened drinks in your diet. But each additional sugar load requires that you exercise a little more to maintain that balance and keep yourself WHealthy. With busy lives, the amount of time most of us have for exercise is limited, so it makes a lot of sense to simply reduce the sugar we drink.

CALORIE CONTENT OF COMMON DRINKS

Drink	Volume	Calories	Exercise Equivalent (Walking, minutes)
Soda	12 ounces	125 - 190	20 - 30
Sweet Bottled Tea	12 ounces	130 - 150	20 - 25
Unsweetened Orange Juice	12 ounces	150 - 180	20 - 25
Sports Drink	12 ounces	85 - 100	10 - 15
Whole Milk	12 ounces	220	30
Nonfat Milk	12 ounces	125	15
Beer	12 ounces	155	25
Light Beer	12 ounces	104	15
Red Wine	5 ounces	125	20
White Wine	5 ounces	125	20
Hard Liquor	1.5 ounces	96	15

THE POWER OF FOOD AND MOOD: COMBAT COMFORT EATING

Food and mood are closely related. When we cry as babies, we are nursed. When we throw temper tantrums in the grocery store as toddlers, we are offered snacks to distract us. When we have a birthday or graduation, we celebrate with a feast. Advertisers reinforce positive association with foods to increase their sales. It's not surprising, then, that when we experience strong emotions, we eat.

Hunger is a powerful physical and chemical stimulus that keeps us alive. Under natural circumstances, that's exactly what it does: keeps us alive. It tells us to eat so that we can have sufficient energy to run our bodies.

There is, however, another form of hunger that interferes with nature's elegant design. Emotional hunger drives *comfort eating*, a destructive behavior that is not responsive to regular feedback and control mechanisms. Comfort eating is not a weakness or simple lack of self-discipline. Instead, it is a psychological reaction that strives to suppress undesirable feelings or fill emotional voids. It is an often-successful, subconscious, short-term coping strategy with disastrous long-term consequences. Our bodies seek instant relief with foods like chocolate that stimulate the release of serotonin in the brain or a rapid, transient spike in blood sugar. After bingeing, though, our emotional hunger rapidly becomes guilt and shame, exaggerating our unresolved emotional needs and precipitating a chronic cycle of negative eating.

There are several major differences between emotional and physical hunger. First, physical hunger is driven by your stomach. When your body needs food, you feel the emptiness and "hunger pangs" in your belly. Emotional hunger, on the other hand, is driven by an emotional need, and the food "craving" is in your head. Second, physical hunger grows steadily as your body sends your brain messages with increasing intensity, driving you to eat. By contrast, emotional hunger tends to arise quickly and demand instant gratification. Third, physical hunger is satisfied by food. It sounds simple, but when the need is met, the hunger goes away. Emotional hunger is not satisfied by food, and you'll notice that the "emptiness" doesn't go away even when you eat. Fourth, physical hunger is satisfied by any food, while emotional hunger is often focused on a specific food (especially fatty or sugar-loaded food). And finally, physical hunger is replaced by a sense of emotional satisfaction after the meal, whereas emotional eating tends to be followed by guilt, shame, and regret.

There are many different causes of emotional hunger. The stress hormone, *cortisol*, provokes food cravings, especially for salty, sweet, and high-fat delicacies. With the prevalence of relationship conflicts, financial pressures, work stress, unemployment, and health problems, this is a common cause of emotional hunger. Eating can also be a way to fill emotional voids and suppress uncomfortable emotions. Comfort eating provides temporary relief from sadness, anxiety, loneliness, and low self-esteem. It can stave off intellectual boredom. A combination of numbing and avoidance briefly silences these painful voices.

Sometimes, comfort eating is habitual. You grab something to eat as you walk in the door, or sit down at your desk to work, or drive. Social pressures can also exaggerate intrinsic tendencies toward comfort eating. Overindulgent friends can exert overt influence, and you may be encouraged to overeat to keep others happy. Similarly, not all comfort eating is the result of sadness. Happiness may trigger similar vulnerability. Sometimes, when we're happy, we reward ourselves excessively with food.

Finally, fatigue has a direct physiological effect on our appetite-suppression (or satiety) system. *Ghrelin* is a hormone that stimulates appetite, the same way that leptin signals the brain to stop eating. Inadequate sleep increases ghrelin and decreases leptin, tipping the scale toward excessive eating.

Emotional eating is characterized by several traits: You eat to feel better. You reward yourself with food. You eat more when you're feeling stressed. You eat when you're not hungry. You regularly eat until you've stuffed yourself. You feel that food has irresistible power over you. You feel guilty after eating.

The best way to address emotional hunger is head-on (pun intended, because the head, not the stomach, is the source of the problem). First, be healthy. Physical activity and relaxation reduce stress and stimulate the release of endorphins that elevate mood. Social engagement is a powerful stimulant of serotonin, which also raises mood. Adequate sleep ensures the appropriate ghrelin/leptin balance.

Second, become a mindful eater. Be aware of your eating habits and preferences. Eat slowly, appreciating rather than gulping your food. This also gives the stretch receptors in the stomach the chance to alert the brain when it is time to stop eating. Recognize the relationship between your mood and your eating habits. When you feel hunger, pause. Ask yourself if this is physical or emotional hunger. It's probably not physical hunger if you don't feel hunger pangs in your stomach. Give the craving time to pass. Slowly drink a large glass of water, then reevaluate.

Self-awareness is the first step in controlling the overeating that comes from emotional hunger. If you encounter emotional hunger often and respond to it with indulgence, then acknowledge that you are a comfort eater. You're not alone. Identify and manage the underlying cause and triggers. It may be a good idea to keep a diary and look for patterns between mood and food. Once you identify the root cause, take steps to address it. Tame your stress. Find other ways to fill the emotional voids and fight boredom: take a walk, call a friend, listen to music, or dance. Learn to accept your feelings—even the bad ones—and love yourself and your body. Avoid temptation. Don't stock comfort foods in your pantry, and don't go the grocery store when you're sad. Be gentle with yourself and learn from setbacks. Forgive yourself quickly and start fresh. Don't chastise yourself. Get right back to affirming thoughts; you're not going to overfeed somebody you love. If you've tried all this and are still struggling, then you may benefit from professional help in identifying and managing the root cause of your emotional eating.

One last trick. When you catch yourself with emotional hunger, say (out loud, if you're brave enough), "I am not really hungry." Permit your cognitive brain to influence your emotional brain, allowing you to wait for physical hunger to return. You will learn a lot more about this technique later in the book.

KEY #3: SLEEP RIGHT

Cultivate sleep for peak performance.

> *"Early to bed and early to rise makes a man healthy, wealthy, and wise."*
>
> BENJAMIN FRANKLIN, POOR RICHARD'S ALMANAC

This quote comes from *Poor Richard's Almanac* (circa 1735), Benjamin Franklin's scientific journal. In it, he foreshadowed truths that modern science continues to unravel (though I would change his word "man" to "person").

As a young physician, I was invited to participate in an unusual event. I was asked to provide medical support to two inspiring young men who were intent on achieving a world record for squash-playing endurance. In reality, they could have been trying to break the world record for sleeplessness. In order to qualify, they had to play through several days and nights, snatching only brief moments of sleep in permitted rest intervals. I forget the actual number of days and hours played, but watching their physical, mental, and emotional responses to sleep deprivation remains one of my most remarkable professional memories. Not for the first time, the experience made me realize the profound value of sleep in our lives.

Why do we sleep? Experts have proposed two major theories. First, sleep allows the body to repair and rejuvenate (the *Restorative Theory*). Growth hormone release, muscle growth, tissue repair, and synthesis of key restorative proteins all occur predominately during sleep. Second, sleep enables structural and organizational development of the brain (the *Brain*

Plasticity Theory). Babies and young children sleep for thirteen to fourteen hours per day to help their brains develop. In contrast, sleep deprivation impairs learning and intellectual performance.

Do we as a society sleep enough? The answer is a resounding *No!* In 1992, concerns about changing sleep habits prompted a study by the National Commission on Sleep Disorders. The report, titled *Wake Up America! A National Sleep Alert,*[19] revealed that Americans were sleeping 20 percent less than we did at the end of the nineteenth century. More recently, this decrease in sleep was estimated to cause almost 40,000 casualties per year. Modern social development has outstripped evolution. We're living at a pace that our bodies have not yet adjusted to, with significant negative results.

And trends have shown that we are continuing to sleep less over time. Data produced by the National Sleep Foundation[20] show that 71 percent

PERCENT OF ADULTS IN THE UNITED STATES WHO USUALLY SLEPT 6 HOURS OR LESS A NIGHT

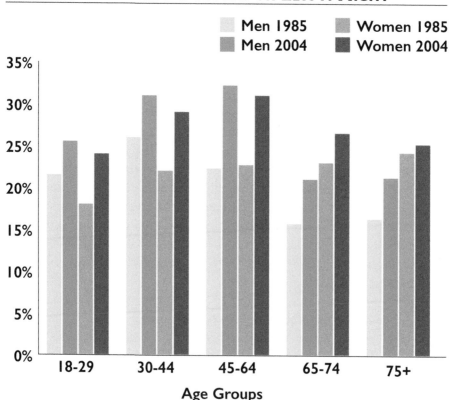

of Americans report getting less than eight hours of sleep on weeknights. More interesting to me is that the number of people reporting lack of sleep is 8 percent higher than it was in the data produced seven years earlier. The chart below comes from CDC data[21] and shows the same trend across all the subgroups evaluated. This is entirely in keeping with the other physical disasters (lack of exercise and obesity) that are the consequence of our (R) evolutionary Gap. In the past, we would go to sleep when the sun set and rise again with daylight. That is no longer the case. Our societal evolution has given us the technology—but not the physiology—to function all the time, anytime…at significant personal cost!

Sleep is the third essential component of BodyWHealth. Adequate sleep helps you fight against the downward physical and mental spiral associated with aging. Inadequate sleep will jeopardize the gains you make by exercising and eating healthy.

WHAT IS HEALTHY SLEEP?

Good, healthy sleep has a pattern. A "normal" night of sleep is characterized by four to five sleep cycles, each lasting about ninety minutes. In each of these cycles, four stages of *slow-wave sleep* (so called because of the slow waves of electrical activity in the brain that occur during that stage) are followed by one period of *Rapid Eye Movement (REM) sleep*. We know that physical and mental restoration occurs during slow-wave sleep, but the function of REM sleep remains largely a mystery. What we do know is

STAGES OF SLEEP

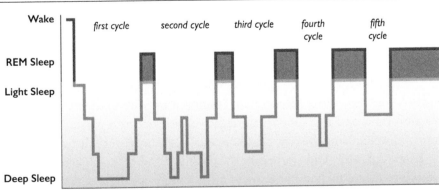

that REM sleep is the phase of sleep in which we dream. It is characterized by intense brain activity, rapid eye movements (with closed eyes), elevated heart rate and breathing, and muscle paralysis that presumably protects us against physical injury that might occur if we acted out our dreams. Adults have up to two hours of REM sleep per night, while infants have much more (as much as 50 percent of their sleep), suggesting that it may be associated with mental development.

The opposite of sleep is alertness. If we engage in normal sleep patterns, we have two daytime alertness peaks: one in the morning, and the other in the late afternoon. These are separated by an early afternoon dip in alertness. I can remember that, for some reason, for me this dip always coincided with my Latin classes in high school!

THE DANGERS OF NOT SLEEPING WELL

Sleep has direct impact on your health, and hence your WHealth. The specific benefits of sleep have been defined indirectly, through studying the impact of sleep deprivation and through observational studies that identify associations between sleep patterns and disease prevalence. Two critical concepts have emerged: *sleep need* and *sleep debt*.

Sleep need is defined as the pressure to go to sleep. It builds from the moment we open our eyes in the morning. We can measure sleep need using levels of a brain chemical called *adenosine*. Substances like caffeine can temporarily mask the effect of adenosine, leaving us less aware of the need for sleep for a short while. Ultimately, however, sleep need is only "reset" by a full night's sleep.

If you don't get enough rest, your sleep need is not reset, and you begin to accumulate sleep debt. A cumulative sleep deficit grows with long-term sleep deprivation. Daytime drowsiness is a warning sign of the accumulation of excessive sleep debt. Cumulative sleep debt has a significant impact on your major bodily systems, with profound negative effect on your WHealth.

In the short term, sleep deprivation results in impaired judgment, reduced reaction time, and bad moods, all negatively impacting a person's ability to function well during the day. This happens with surprisingly little reduction in sleep quantity, and surprisingly quickly. Studies have demonstrated neurological and mental impairment after a single all-nighter that is similar to having a blood alcohol level of 0.05 percent—a level that's considered legally intoxicated. Loss of as little as one and a half hours of sleep on a single night can reduce daytime alertness by as much as 30 percent (as any parent of young children knows). This reduced daytime performance includes both impaired memory and impaired cognitive functions. After limited sleep deprivation, only attention and working (short-term) memory are affected, but after prolonged sleep loss, long-term memory and decision-making skills are also impaired. All of these impairments result in a significant increase in all sorts of personal risk, with higher rates of car accidents, occupational injuries, and relationship problems.

Over the long term, sleep deprivation results in a long list of serious medical conditions, the greatest of which is premature death. A study[22] published in 2010 in the journal *Sleep* found the risk of death to be four times greater in men who slept less than six hours per night compared with those who slept more than six hours per night. In addition to this alarming finding, sleep deprivation has also been associated with an increased risk of stress-related illness, major depression and alcohol abuse, heart disease, high blood pressure, stroke, obesity, and diabetes.

One of the serious consequences of long-term sleep deprivation is that it undermines your immune system. Early interest in this topic started when scientists noticed that both sick animals and sick humans often chose to sleep. I grew up in an era when it was not unexpected for us to get measles, mumps, chicken pox, and several other viruses that are largely prevented by immunization today. Apart from the fever, I can remember going to bed each time I got sick and sleeping for many hours as my body fought the infection. There is some evidence in animal research to suggest that animals also have a better chance of surviving severe bacterial infections if they are allowed to sleep for long periods of time.

The scientific community is increasingly aware of an association between sleep debt and cancer. This seems logical given that the immune system plays such a strong role in protecting against cancer, and that lack of sleep weakens the immune system. Recent research has shown a link between sleep deprivation and the prevalence of colon cancer.[23] Another study showed that women who developed aggressive breast cancer and had a high rate of tumor recurrence had slept fewer hours in the period that led up to their cancer diagnosis than those who developed less aggressive breast cancer and had a low rate of tumor recurrence.[24]

Clearly, the impact of sleep on the immune system can be either devastating or life-saving. Sleep is not a luxury activity. It is an essential part of life, and like breathing, you should do it often and do it well!

The Link Between Sleep Deprivation and Obesity

By now you know that excess fat facilitates systemic inflammation, which in turn promotes many of the nasty diseases we worry about today, like heart disease, diabetes, and even cancer. Sleep debt has been demonstrated to increase appetite, favor energy storage as fat, and activate genes that cause obesity. On the other hand, healthy long-term sleep habits protect you and your health in several important ways.

First, sleep helps to reduce belly fat. Poor sleep drives stress and anxiety, which both contribute directly to the buildup of body fat. The stress hormone cortisol not only drives body fat accumulation, but it also increases appetite. Then, sleep deprivation diminishes the body's sensitivity to insulin, a hormone in the blood that regulates the processing of sugar for energy. If insulin sensitivity is reduced, the body takes more fat from the blood and packs it away into your fat stores. Stress and anxiety also often disrupt our exercise routines. This combination of high calorie intake, low calorie burn rate, and a metabolism that favors fat storage drives weight gain, especially in the form of dangerous belly fat. In fact, studies have shown that dieters who sleep badly lose half as much weight as those who sleep well, despite having the same calorie intake.[25]

Sleep also helps you eat less. People deprived of sleep eat 300 to 500 calories per day more than when they are well rested, and they also choose unhealthier foods that are higher in saturated fats.[26] In the previous chapter we learned about the delicate balance between two opposing hormones that control our appetite: ghrelin (the appetite stimulant) and leptin (the fullness alerter). Poor sleep disrupts the balance and regular rhythm[27] of both hormones. In particular, it increases the levels of ghrelin and reduces the levels of leptin,[28] driving excess eating. In addition to these metabolic effects, sleep deprivation leaves us susceptible to poor dietary decision-making. Research has shown that we eat bigger portions and select poorer-quality meals when we are tired. Tiredness sensitizes our reward centers, so we experience more food cravings when our sleep quality is poor.

Finally, sleep helps to suppress obesity genes. Some people have a genetic predisposition to obesity, and those obesity genes require specific circumstances to activate them. Studies of twins have shown beyond doubt that sleep deprivation helps switch on the obesity genes.[29] Twins have identical DNA, so both siblings in each pair being studied had the same genetic predisposition to obesity. But the twins who slept less were heavier than their well-rested siblings. Clearly, we have much to be gained by sleeping well.

Your Prescription for WHealth

Healthy sleep is a critical component of BodyWHealth. It drives mental, emotional, and physical health for any WHealth Seeker. That is why the third Key to WHealth is to *cultivate sleep for peak performance.* This will help you to retain your youth for longer. For most of us, this means sleeping more than we currently do.

What is the right amount of sleep? We don't have a perfect generalizable recommendation because sleep need is highly individualized; however, it is generally recommended that adults sleep a minimum of seven to eight hours every night for optimal mental function. We do know that less than six hours of sleep per day[30] has been shown to result in significant mental impairment. The risk of serious accident is clearly increased at this level, regardless of other negative impacts. In the same study of sleep deprivation and neurological function, subjects who slept eight hours a day performed very well.

The best way to determine how much sleep *you* need is by tracking your level of alertness throughout the day. It's rather simple, actually: When you struggle with drowsiness during the day, it means that you need to sleep more at night. After a lifetime of research, Professor William Dement, one of the world's leading sleep researchers and a renowned professor at Stanford University, summed up his findings in a single piece of pragmatic advice. He suggests that we should "sleep until you can't sleep any more."

SIMPLE RECOMMENDATIONS FOR SLEEPING RIGHT

1. *Value sleep.* You must understand the value of sleep and defend it as an important part of your life.

2. *Sleep enough.* Sleep enough to stay alert during the day. This will help you to retain your youth for longer. For most of us, this means sleeping more than we currently do.

3. *Relax.* Even if you're having trouble going to sleep, don't get angry with yourself. Lie quietly with your eyes closed. Breathe deeply and let yourself relax. You're resting, and that's a good thing, even if you lie awake a little while!

4. *Remain still.* Get up if you need a drink or the bathroom, but don't become too active. Movement alerts sensors in your joints that it is time for wakefulness. This sends signals to your brain, and again, you disrupt your circadian (sleep) rhythm. Lie quietly.

5. *Use the dark.* Don't put on the lights. They send a signal to your brain that it's daytime and can disrupt your circadian rhythm.

6. *Turn off electronics.* The blue light emitted by electronic screens and many night-lights suppresses the secretion of *melatonin*, a hormone that regulates your circadian rhythm and is important to the quality of your sleep. You're not doing yourself a favor if you're absorbed in your computer, tablet, or smartphone when you go to bed. Similarly, don't grab them after waking prematurely if you're hoping to fall back asleep quickly. If you have to have night-lights, go for red—it's the least disruptive color to melatonin secretion.

7. *Use a book.* If you really need to do something to help you unwind before bed, then read a book. Don't use a bright light; dim light is better. Do you remember trying to stay awake while you had to study? It can be difficult. Reading has a soothing effect on the brain, and ideally your eyelids will start drooping.

8. ***Don't snack at night.*** Most of the things you grab from the fridge will result in a sugar surge, which will wake you up. It's also likely to keep your brain awake for a little while before your insulin kicks in to reduce the level of blood sugar again.

9. ***Take advantage of alertness.*** Use your daytime alertness peaks wisely. They are your most productive times!

10. ***Get help if you need it.*** If you have severe sleep disruption, consult your physician. Before you grab for a bottle of sleeping tablets, though, consider other options, such as cognitive behavioral therapy,[31] which has been shown in several research studies to be better than our strongest sleep drugs.

CONCLUSION

Sleep is one of the three critical elements of Mother Nature's primal design, and it is vital for your health and happiness. Each day, we must balance work and rest. When we sleep, the army of rejuvenation engages, reversing the damage of the day, restoring us and keeping us young. Ignoring Mother Nature's intent invokes disastrous physical and emotional consequences. Honoring your primal design by cultivating healthy sleep habits unlocks both physical and emotional WHealth. Sleep well. This is the road to abundance.

In addition to sleeping enough to stay alert all day, I advocate that you take advantage of another potentially uplifting benefit sleep has to offer: dreams.

THE POWER OF DREAMS: UNIFYING YOUR COGNITIVE AND EMOTIONAL BRAINS

Did you ever have a dream that changed your life? Did you ever wake in the middle of the night, drenched with sweat and filled with terror? Did you ever jump out of bed to check on a loved one? Did you ever try to force yourself back to sleep because you were enjoying a dream so much that you didn't ever want to wake up?

No discussion of sleep is complete without some reference to dreams, although candidly, it is very hard to make any connections between dreams and health or happiness—other than to say that when you are happy, you tend to have more happy dreams than unhappy ones! I'll share what we know about dreams, as well as a couple of suggestions for how you might derive some benefit from them.

Sleep researchers devote time to studying brain waves and other metabolic activities during sleep, and then force dreamers into wakefulness, prompting them to recall the content of their nocturnal journeys. Psychologists and anthropologists work to relate dreams to psychosocial events and needs. Spiritualists look for messages in dreams. Not surprisingly, there is little consensus among these groups, and large knowledge gaps exist in this profoundly moving aspect of our lives. The divergence of opinion is not really surprising, as the alternative reality of dreams is very hard to research.

Scientists agree that dreaming happens mainly during REM sleep. In this phase of sleep, the entire body is paralyzed except for the eye muscles. Some believe that sleep paralysis is designed to protect the dreamer, who otherwise might act out the vivid dreams, sometimes with disastrous results. A group of scientists has explored the similarities between sleep paralysis and the deep trance-like state (called the "tonic immobility reflex") some animals enter when "playing dead" as a defense mechanism. This tonic immobility reflex is the last refuge of certain species that fake death to escape predators. While the paralysis humans experience during REM sleep is physiologically similar to the tonic immobility reflex, it's hard to prove an evolutionary link between the two. What is clear about REM sleep is that the unparalyzed eyes appear to react to the dream as though it was real. The eyes scan and follow the action being played out in the theater of the sleeping brain.

There is far less agreement about what dreams actually are, and why we have them in the first place. A prominent group of neuroscientists believe that dreams are nothing more than a collection of random nerve activity in the brain. I find this theory hard to substantiate given the colorful stories I have experienced personally in many of my dreams. Modern psychologists believe that dreams either reflect issues we are currently wrestling with (the *emotional processing theory*) or serve to prepare us for events that may occur in the future (the *threat simulation theory*). To unite these hypotheses, other scientists propose that our brains react to the random nerve activity to give it meaning. It may be that our current emotional and psychological context serves as a filter, ensuring that our brains apply relevant interpretations. For now, the final answer eludes us.

Throughout history, we have attempted to interpret the meaning of dreams. Many of us will be familiar with the biblical story of Joseph interpreting Pharaoh's dreams as it is presented in the Tim Rice and Andrew Lloyd Webber musical *Joseph and The Amazing Technicolor Dreamcoat*. Joseph found favor with Pharaoh because he had the magical ability to interpret the ruler's dreams for him. You can pay modern-day Josephs good money to interpret your dreams for you, too.

Professor William Dement, the grandfather of modern sleep science, reminds us to differentiate between the *meaning* of a dream and its *purpose*. To date, we have no definitive scientific conclusion on either. This gives us broad scope in deciding what to make of dreams, and I have a few suggestions to guide you on your sleepy way.

First, enjoy dreams! You have roughly two hours of REM sleep on an average night, and you dream during all of it. That means you get to watch one full-length movie, or perhaps four sitcoms, every night! You remember a dream when you waken during the REM phase in which you were dreaming.

This happens when the emotional weight of the experience exceeds your sleepiness. We know from nuclear scans of the brain that your emotional brain and long-term memory centers are hyperactive during dreams, while other centers such as sensory and computational regions are passive. This explains the remarkable phenomenon of waking with your cognitive brain aware that what you just experienced was *not* real, while your emotional brain firmly believes it *was* real. This suggests to me that the cognitive brain served up a lifelike experience to the emotional brain for good reason.

Which takes me to my second recommendation: Use dreams! Use them to help you interpret and understand issues you are dealing with in your day-to-day life. In a way, your body puts your brain onto the therapist's couch every night. Observe, learn, and grow. Don't get caught up in doom and gloom forecasts. No science has ever demonstrated that dreams foreshadow reality. What we do know is that visualization is a powerful tool when you're awake. So, use the equally powerful theater of the mind while you're asleep to prepare you for the future. In the next section of this book, we will discuss the power of belief. To *believe*, you need to couple the efforts of the cognitive and emotional brains harmoniously behind an *idea*, which becomes a *desire*, and finally an invincible *belief* that overcomes doubt and leads to success. Embrace the moments when you wake in ecstasy, with the cognitive and emotional brains in deep alignment. Use this force to drive success in your life.

I am reminded of the great dream that Dr. Martin Luther King, Jr., American pastor and human rights activist, shared with the world on August 28, 1963. I believe that he had a real dream, a dream in which his cognitive and emotional brains were so tightly aligned that success was inevitable. I recommend that you read or listen to his deeply moving words, and ask yourself if dreams can come true. Then close your eyes, find your own desires, arm them with belief, and build your WHealthy future!

THE DARK MENACE: STRESS

Manage your stress wisely.

Hans Selye, considered by many to be the first scientist to demonstrate the biological response to stress, once said, "It is not stress that kills us. It is our reaction to it."

You will read about stress in almost every popular magazine that you pick up today. Each generation seems to have boasted the highest stress levels in history. While stress is hard to measure objectively, I think there is some validity in this claim over recent years. I don't believe that the stress of *individual* major life events is any higher today than it was 100 years ago. In fact, given our greater medical proficiency, we may actually encounter fewer health stresses than prior generations. But most would probably agree that the pace of modern life has escalated the *volume* of stressors significantly. We no longer wait for surface mail to bring problems to our attention. They arrive continuously in our email inboxes, and demand immediate resolution.

This is caused by the same fundamental problem that threatens our WHealth in other ways: the (R)evolutionary Gap. Technological progress has vastly outpaced our biological evolution. Today we face an avalanche of stimuli that induce stress, but we have not yet had time for adaptations in our physical constitution that enable us to manage the consequences of those stimuli.

Stress may be the most explicit example of the deep interrelationship between body and mind. In everyday language, we tend to use the term "stress" somewhat ambiguously, to describe both a negative situation that triggers discomfort and our anticipation or response to such an event. We could probably more accurately call these painful situations "distress." You will see a little later that (limited) stress is healthy. It is an adaptive response that prepares our body to handle the challenges of living. When you go beyond the healthy, however, *stress* becomes *distress*.

The challenges of our early ancestors were mainly physical and short-lived. They had to run to escape from danger and to catch their food, and they had to fight to protect themselves. Nature ensured that early humans had rapid response systems that mobilized their internal resources to cope with these transient crises. When faced with imminent danger, their bodies released two critical hormones, *adrenaline* and cortisol, to kick-start their physiology into action mode and mobilize the energy they needed to respond vigorously. After the flurry of action (assuming they survived), the temporary physiological disruption abated, with no lasting unwanted consequences. The system worked well.

Today, our stressors are very different. Very few of our crises are physical in nature. We seldom need to fight or take flight. When we do, our body still works beautifully. We release adrenaline and cortisol. These hormones are put to good use, and our bodies respond with a burst of activity. The system resets quickly afterward, as designed, with no lasting consequences.

But the vast majority of stressful stimuli that we modern men and women face are mental or emotional in nature, meaning we have no need to fight or flee. Moreover, given our advanced cognitive abilities, it is often the *anticipation* of possible danger that triggers our physical stress response more than actual danger. Add to this the sheer volume of stress that we cope with on a daily basis and the sleep deprivation that impairs our ability to recover between stressful days, and we quickly advance into the territory of chronic stress overload. Again, the (R)evolutionary Gap rears its ugly head. The rapid pace of societal transformation has outstripped our body's ability to adapt. Instead of working with a new, improved rapid response system 2.0—which we have yet to develop—we must cope with this new and different stress landscape with the original version of the rapid response system. This is a huge problem for WHealth Seekers.

Today, our busy day, or the thought of financial ruin, or the anticipation of being laid off still triggers release of the same two hormones, adrenaline and cortisol. But we don't run away or turn and fight with our bodies. We don't use these hormones to good effect. Instead, they flood our system with chemicals we don't need or use, which prepare our bodies for physical encounters that don't happen. This has significant cumulative negative consequences.

Adrenaline activates the cardiovascular system. For fight or flight, we need to have our heart and lungs pumping maximally to circulate oxygen to our furiously working muscles. When the threat is physical, and we actually have to break into a run, this physiological turbo boost is appropriate. Unfortunately, our body goes through this same preparation even with mental and emotional stress, when we don't need the same cardiovascular response. Under these circumstances, chronic stress invites serious health risks like high blood pressure and heart disease.

Cortisol plays a more subtle role in this process; its negative impact is mainly on systems that you should be well familiar with by now: the inflammatory and immune systems. Excess cortisol, the result of prolonged stress, has a sinister impact on our inflammatory balance. It suppresses the inflammatory cytokines. The problem is that its most profound impact is on the beneficial cytokines, the anti-inflammatory cytokines. Remember that this group, led by IL10, is the force of rejuvenation that works against decay to keep us young. So, stress compounds the systemic inflammatory overload we have from our sedentary lifestyle and excess of visceral body fat, increasing our risk of developing heart disease, diabetes, and cancer.

Cortisol also suppresses the immune system. A recurrent elevation in cortisol, which is a result of chronic stress, impedes our immune army, making us vulnerable to infection and cancer. Not only do we develop more infections, but it also takes us longer to recover from them. Our immune armies are less capable of fighting established cancers, and our immune surveillance is weakened, so our bodies overlook early cancers more easily, allowing them to establish themselves.

To make matters worse, when we are stressed, we tend to eat more and exercise less. This compounds our disastrous pro-inflammatory, weakened immune system leaning even further. It's a powerful recipe for trouble.

Thus, our ancient design leaves us only modestly equipped to cope with the stresses of the modern era. We remain well suited to physical danger, but a surplus of adrenaline and cortisol, the consequence of omnipresent mental and emotional distress, have a significant negative impact on our health and happiness.

STRESS, DISTRESS, AND THE OVERTRAINING SYNDROME

As you read this book, you may be feeling *tired, jaded, stale, fatigued,* or *burned out*. That may even be the reason that you chose to read this book in the first place. These are all common terms used to describe the physical and emotional consequences of *overwork*. Competitive athletes experience the same outcome when they *overtrain*, and we can learn a lot about how to handle overwork from research conducted in this special group of high performers. How can you prevent and, if necessary, recover from this debilitating state?

Stress is actually a positive force. Without it, we would neither perform nor grow. If you study the normal performance curve below, you will notice how increasing your workload improves your performance. Stress plays a vital role in driving your accomplishments—up to a point. But the law of diminishing returns kicks in at some stage, and additional effort produces less improvement in performance. Most important to this concept is the balance of work (or training) and recovery. Athletes know this well. They stress their muscles during training in order to make them stronger, but they *must* allow them time to recover and rebuild before re-stressing them. That's true for our brains and psyches, too: Sleeping or resting too little impairs their performance. Each of us must find our own highly individualized optimal ratio of work to rest that drives us to sustainable peak performance.

So, it's easy right? Work harder and harder, and then when things start going wrong, back off and find your "zone"? That is true to some extent, but it's not so easy, actually. The problem, as you can see below, is that at the far right of the performance curve is a giant cliff. You step over the edge at your peril. It's a long, painful ride to the bottom, and the way back up is excruciating. The most useful thing you can learn to do is to push yourself as close as possible to the cliff without actually falling off the edge. Here's the problem, though: Our scientific insight is poor at best when it comes to providing guidance in this endeavor. In my personal experience, most elite athletes have fallen off the cliff at least once. That's probably also true for anybody who is particularly driven at work. We are determined to give the max. That's a respectable instinct as long as we understand the consequences.

The good thing about the edge is that there *may* be warning signs before you get there. Notice that I said "may." Unfortunately, again, the science is not strong enough for me to say unequivocally that there *are* warning signs.

THE PERFORMANCE CURVE

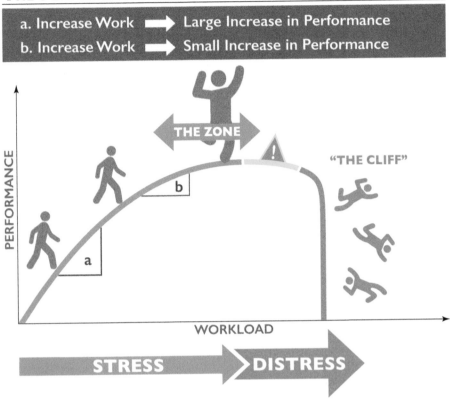

Be aware, you may suddenly fall off the edge, even if you are super-diligent in listening to your body. I'd say that this is pretty rare, though, and that the majority of those who report falling off the cliff unexpectedly didn't listen that carefully to, or even ignored, important warning signs.

Here is the science about the warning zone. This is the zone where *stress* becomes *distress*, implying that you begin to experience physical, emotional, and/or psychological discomfort. Sleep disruption is often the most common symptom; it may manifest as difficulty in falling asleep, increased wakefulness through the night, or reduced quality of sleep. All of these sleep issues result in you feeling tired when you wake up. You can imagine a negative cycle developing rapidly, where overtraining results in sleep disruption that in turn impairs performance. Competitive people react by increasing their workload to offset the poor performance, precipitating a downward spiral. This is the quick route off the cliff!

The other physical measure that regularly alerts us to overtraining is resting heart rate. A gradual upward creep in resting heart rate with no other cause (such as an underlying infection) is a strong warning signal. I advise all elite athletes I work with to track their waking heart rate. Your waking heart rate is your heart rate as you wake, before any of the noise of the day can influence your cardiac rhythm. I'd bet that resting heart rate is good at detecting burnout in non-athletes, too!

There are other diagnostic tests for overtraining, but these are not sufficiently reliable to receive broad support from medical scientists. We know that cortisol, the body's stress hormone, tends to drop as you burn out. The adrenal system, responsible for your fight and flight reactions, becomes fatigued and under-responsive. In athletes, *glutamine* (involved with cellular energy metabolism and protein synthesis), *glutamate* (important for healthy nerve function), and *testosterone* (a driver of muscle growth and recovery) all tend to be reduced in the overtraining syndrome.

It is interesting that athletes experience reduced perceptions of strength and recovery when they are overtrained. In truth, the overtrained athlete can actually do more work than they think they can, but the brain chooses to underreach, protecting the body from further injury. This explains the

THE PERFORMANCE CURVE DANGER ZONE

When you are working or training in the danger zone, a trivial insult like a minor illness brings the cliff closer, possibly with dire consequences.

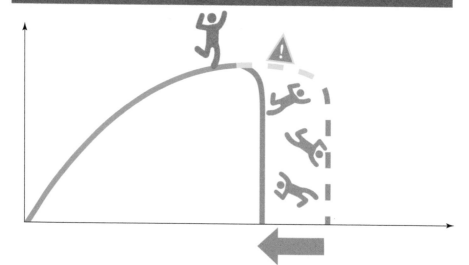

THE PERFORMANCE CURVE RECOVERY PATH

The long walk is the only recovery path for most, often after a recuperation phase!

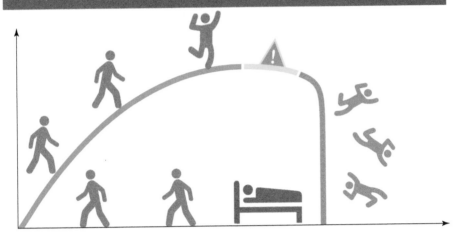

extraordinary fatigue associated with long-term stress. When you're burning the candle at both ends, your body attempts to protect itself. It tries to get you to take your foot off the gas pedal, even though it has more gas in the tank. The sensation of overwhelming fatigue is a warning signal. Heed it!

Perhaps the biggest danger while you're in the warning zone is that a relatively small stress can nudge you over the edge. You may be aware that you are in the danger zone, but feel confident because of the fact that you are aware of how close you are to the edge; then something small and unexpected suddenly throws you off the cliff. The final stress may be, for example, a minor illness or a personal disappointment that brings the cliff closer toward you—and over you go!

Now here is the bad news: Only a tiny minority is able to grab hold of the steep cliff on the way down to immediately climb their way back up. For the most part, it's a quick, painful descent to the bottom, with the only way back a long walk up your original pathway, often requiring a convalescent period before that climb is possible. Burnout can be disastrous. People with noble intentions and an exceptional work ethic can find themselves collapsed in a heap at the bottom of the cliff. It can take months, even years, before they find the appetite for hard work again. It can be a very long and painful journey back up the performance curve.

The best approach is prevention. Listen very carefully to your body. Push through minor resistance, but listen for persistent warnings. Track your sleep. Track your resting (waking) heart rate. Nobody knows your body like you do, and everybody's performance curve is unique (and can change over time). Superhuman ideation is both dangerous and arrogant. If you hear warning signs, back up a little; reduce your workload and increase your rest and recovery. And then back up some more. You need to have some reserve for the unexpected. If you do this, you *should* be able to keep yourself in your zone. That's where you find health, happiness, and prosperity. That's where you find BodyWHealth!

BREATHING: YOUR SOURCE OF POWER

Long-term stress erodes BodyWHealth. It induces a physiological state that impairs performance and increases the risk of disease. But one little trick can have surprising benefits in managing stress.

What's the first thing we all do when we enter the world? What's the last thing we all do as we exit? You got it? That's right. We breathe. We fill our lungs with oxygen. Even before letting out the first cry to announce our arrival immediately after birth, we take a deep breath. Breathing is that rhythmic, mystical process by which we bring in life-giving oxygen to drive our bodies and brains. It's also the means of eliminating life's toxic by-products. When we do it well, we thrive. When we do it poorly, we suffer.

The pivotal role that breathing plays in our lives is captured in many phrases and idioms. Before we start a daunting task, we say, "Take a deep breath." We wait "with baited breath" for important news. If we surprise somebody, we "take their breath away."

Subconscious reflexes control breathing. Breathing in, otherwise known as *inspiration*, is an active process driven by the diaphragm and chest muscles. Breathing out, or *expiration*, is passive; the lung collapses using elastic recoil. The nerve center that controls breathing is situated at the base of your brain, a highly protected region of your body, because breathing is so critically important to life. Chemical receptors detect the concentration of carbon dioxide in your blood. If it rises to a certain level, your body stimulates you to breathe. Interestingly, you have the ability to override the autopilot on your breathing function. This makes breathing unlike the body's other automated functions.

Two major components of your central nervous system control your breathing. The *sympathetic nervous system* is responsible for spurring you into action, provoking the "fight or flight" response that is critical for survival. Your ancestors had to run to eat and to escape being eaten. When the sympathetic nerves fire, you increase your respiratory rate, pumping your lungs to supply more oxygen to fight or take flight. It becomes hard to fill your lungs when you work them so fast; your breathing becomes shallower. The opposite response is driven by the *parasympathetic nervous system*. When these nerve signals dominate, you are lulled into deep relaxation. Your breathing becomes slow and deep. In this state, your metabolic demand for oxygen is low, and your lungs default to deep, rhythmic breathing.

As early humans, we fired up our sympathetic systems for short bursts only. We needed to dash for cover, or sprint to catch the ostrich for dinner. Modern living places a totally different demand on us. The stress of daily living induces long-term low-level activation of stress hormones, triggering tense muscles, a hyper-alert mental state, and (you guessed it!) shallow, rapid breathing. Stress expresses itself very directly in our breathing.

Think of some of the worst moments of your life. Stuck in traffic. Working seven-day weeks to meet a looming deadline. Arguing with a loved one. In each of these situations, your brain pumps out signals to activate your body and focus your mind. You may find your pulse racing. You can feel the tension in your body, especially in your chest and neck muscles. If you observe closely, you will notice that you almost splint your chest, holding it rigid as a wooden barrel; your breathing is shallow and rapid. These are appropriate reactions designed to cope with emergencies, but when we maintain this heightened physiological state over a prolonged period of time, we can trigger serious health and behavioral consequences.

Understanding this science affords us authority over our breathing, and thus over our stress. Unlike other automated bodily functions, we can actively control our breathing. By enforcing a pattern of slow, deep breathing, which the body associates with relaxation, we are able to counteract the impact of stress. I learned almost by accident to use this to calm my children when they had fallen and injured themselves. Even though they're grown, they still laugh at me today. "In through your nose; out through your mouth," they chant when somebody hurts themselves. I carried this through into my medical practice and try to remember it in my personal life when stress gets the upper hand. In through your nose; out through your mouth!

Breath control becomes a powerful means of managing stress. With practice and experience, you will be able to control your breathing, slowing it and deepening it, counteracting your stress. Through this intervention alone, you will be able to shift your unhealthy physiological responses toward more balanced, positive ones. Not only will you be healthier, but you will also be better able to manage the problems that tightened you up in the first place.

One of the pioneers of mind-body medicine is Dr. Herbert Benson of Harvard Medical School and the Massachusetts General Hospital. He described the "relaxation response," the opposite of the fight and flight response. He and many other scientists have demonstrated the central role that breathing plays in inducing the relaxation response. In the short term, we know that relaxation produces a reduction in heart rate and blood pressure, as well as affecting oxygen consumption and brain function. We also know that relaxation affects the actions of our genes. In the presence of relaxation, they instruct our bodies to produce proteins that enhance energy metabolism and immune function, and they suppress the production of a protein that plays a prominent role in inflammation. And as you're probably aware by now, excessive inflammation is at the root of many vexing health problems, including heart disease, diabetes, cancer, and aging.

Now that you know that healthy breathing, even in the absence of disease, is of physiological and functional benefit, what should you do about it? Breathe deep, of course!

SIMPLE RECOMMENDATIONS FOR MANAGING YOUR BREATH AND REDUCING STRESS

1. *Be mindful.* Notice your deep, healing breathing when you are relaxed. When you are tense, notice that you hold your chest, neck, and shoulders tight. Your goal is to consciously calm your breathing, making it slower and deeper at times of stress.

2. *Use your diaphragm.* Babies start out by breathing with their belly. We shift over time to shallow chest breathing. At least 70 percent of the work of adult breathing should be done with your diaphragm. This huge muscle drives your chest like a bellows. Gas exchange is more efficient in the lower airways, so use your belly to suck air deep into your lungs. It also helps lymphatic drainage from the entire body and reduces pressure in your vascular system, thereby reducing the physical effects of stress!

3. *Breathe in through your nose.* Your nasal passages are designed to prepare the air optimally for your lungs. The nose filters impurities and humidifies the air, thus keeping the delicate mucus membranes of your lungs warm and moist.

4. *Exercise.* Have you ever noticed how exercise takes control of your breathing? It's good for other reasons, too. You have to increase your breathing rate to exercise. More importantly, take advantage of the recovery period. When the metabolic demands of your body decline, force your breathing back down to the long, slow, abdominal breathing pattern that is healthy for you and indicates low stress, rather than the nasty, shallow, stressed breathing you had before you went for your exercise.

5. *Sit and stand up straight.* By hunching over, you force the contents of your abdominal cavity up against your diaphragm, inhibiting abdominal breathing. Not only do you feel better and breathe better, but you also feel less stressed when you attend to your posture.

6. *Practice healthy breathing.* You want to concentrate on exhalation, prolonging it to empty your lungs fully while simultaneously draining the stress from your body. Follow this with a deep abdominal breath that fills your lungs and body with oxygen and life. And repeat.

CONCLUSION

I will never forget a lesson taught to me by a very tough, but very kind, horseback-riding instructor. I was training on a new horse, fresh from the plains of the Midwest. He was strong and energetic, but unschooled. I had been thrown from his back twice as I tried to force him over four-foot jumps. To add insult to injury, Ardeth (the riding instructor) yelled at me from across the arena with the most elementary advice: "Roddy, you're not breathing! Why are you not breathing?" In that painful moment, I realized how powerful it was to breathe. As I filled my lungs deeply, I relaxed my shoulders and arms. My hands became gentle on the reins, alleviating the pain in the horse's mouth. I sat low in the saddle, following the horse's movements with my own body, as though we were one. My legs released their vice-like grip on the belly of the horse. The horse's body relaxed, and he broke into a smooth, even canter as we sailed around the course.

What was true for me in the saddle is true for us all in life!

THE PRIMARY ASPIRATION: YOUTH

Enjoy and appreciate your youthfulness.

As bodybuilder Sam (Sonny) Bryant, Jr., said at the age of seventy, "I've met a lot of young guys older than me."

There is a youthfulness to BodyWHealth—more than just the perception of youthfulness that comes from health alone. The pursuit of BodyWHealth invokes physical, mental, and emotional change that opposes the forces of degeneration and decay. If you sit around and do nothing about it, you are destined for decay, even as you live! The good news is that you can do better than this. The same simple interventions that enhance WHealth also drive longevity. Please take the time to *live* in WHealth and *believe* in your youthfulness!

You can't change your birth certificate, just as you cannot cheat your actual age. But you absolutely can live in a younger, healthier, happier body. I'll show you the science, but as importantly, I can tell you that I am truly younger today than when I started this journey. I wish that experience for you, too.

THE SCIENCE OF AGING

Scientists debate the precise cause of aging. It is likely that no single factor is responsible. We know that there are both genetic and environmental factors at work. While scientists are interested in the details of each theory, we ultimately just want to know what to do to live long and healthy lives.

By now you know that an age-related increase in inflammation is intricately linked with many of the diseases we fear, such as heart disease, stroke, diabetes, and cancer. Independent of these diseases, systemic inflammatory overload is also thought to be responsible for the underlying aging process. How does inflammation affect our longevity?

A great deal of work has recently focused on the role of our genes in aging, essentially confirming the presence of the so-called "biological clock." It turns out that you have critical components of your DNA known as *telomeres* that determine your longevity. Telomeres are DNA segments that punctuate the end of your chromosomes (the DNA strands that house your genes). They play a critical role in keeping you young.

Cells are the microscopic building blocks of your body. Wear and tear damages your cells. To stay young, you build new cells to replace the old and defective ones. Each time you create a new cell, you must replicate your DNA, giving the new cell its own little package of genetic material. The problem is that each time you replicate your DNA, you use up a minute fraction of the telomere. When you use up the telomere completely, DNA replication can no longer happen. You are then unable to create new cells, and your body begins decaying faster than it can be rebuilt. It's not hard to see how this accelerates aging; telomeres act like the burning fuse of the age time bomb!

You can see how the size of your telomeres affects your longevity. The longer the telomere, the longer you can replicate DNA to build new cells, and the longer you postpone the inevitable decay of aging. We inherit telomere length from our parents, so there is a good correlation between your parents' longevity and your own. But inflammation has been shown to accelerate telomere dysfunction.[32] Yes, it's back! Not only does inflammation precipitate the long list of diseases we fear, but it causes aging, too—independent of the disease process! Happily, reducing our systemic inflammatory overload both keeps our telomeres functioning well, thereby prolonging our lives, and reduces the likelihood of developing nasty diseases.

Recently, scientists have become excited by animal research that suggests that substantial calorie restriction prolongs life.[33] There is evidence that this reduces systemic inflammation[34] and may have a direct effect on preserving telomere length.[35] There isn't sufficient evidence yet for us to recommend severe calorie restriction in humans, but the observation reinforces my belief in counting calories. We understand now that we can slow the aging process.

One of the major hazards of living is the accumulation of what are called *oxidative free radicals*. I've always liked this term. Although it primarily describes their chemical function, it creates an image of a sinister underground movement: a gang of roving bad guys. Free radicals are the end products of normal biological processes. They are harmful chemicals that damage our genes and tissues. Free-radical-induced damage to our structural tissue results in many of the physical changes we associate with aging, including joint stiffness, skin and bone weakening, and "hardening" of our arteries (and, by the way, cancer[36]). In addition to causing this structural harm, free radicals also damage our *mitochondria*, the tiny intracellular organelles that are responsible for energy metabolism. Disruption of mitochondrial function has a far-reaching impact on other biological processes that all depend on good energy supply. Left unchecked, free radicals go about their destructive business, accelerating the decay of aging.

Fortunately, Mother Nature has designed a system that protects us against free radicals. Healthy cells contain *antioxidants* that round up and neutralize free radicals. When we are young, we have abundant antioxidant supplies that protect us against these nasty toxins. Our intrinsic antioxidant capacity declines with age, possibly (surprise!) related to systemic inflammatory overload. The accumulation of free radicals then activates pro-inflammatory genes,[37] further fueling the inflammatory overload, resulting in a vicious degenerative cycle and accelerated aging.

The good news, as you already know, is that we can limit the excessive inflammation associated with both aging and disease. Exercise reduces the long-term buildup of harmful inflammation and stimulates healthy anti-inflammatory chemicals. Fat cells encourage pro-inflammatory metabolism, so controlling weight is critical to countering the inflammation of aging. BodyWHealth's first two Keys mandate these healthy steps. The same Keys that unlock health also unlock youth! That's the beauty of BodyWHealth.

Anticipating a longer life, we should now think about optimizing our additional years. I know many people who will groan if I tell them that they will live longer. They will picture more years spent in decay. They will worry that we have prolonged the degenerative experience. Not so. I strongly urge that you spend this extra time *living!* We will all age. I want to age gracefully. To me, this means retaining my health, mental function, mobility, happiness, and ability to contribute to the world.

We worry about the mental degeneration commonly associated with age. Again, the news is good, and studies have definitively shown that regular exercise protects our minds. We know that cognitive function declines more slowly in people who exercise regularly.[38] The benefit starts early. In a study that examined people's cognitive function in relation to their fitness status twenty-five years earlier, the researchers found conclusive evidence that people who exercised regularly enjoyed better cognitive function than their more sedentary peers.[39]

Exercise not only delivers this broad array of physical benefits; it also enhances mood. Exercise stimulates the release of hormones that enhance your mood, endorphins and serotonin (the "feel-good" hormones in the brain) in particular. In addition to improving your health and mobility as you age, you can also elevate your mood, so you *are* younger and you *feel* younger.

CONCLUSION

Centuries of people have sought the secret to perpetual youth. With BodyWHealth, enduring youthfulness can be yours! When you treat your body well through exercise, energy balance, quality sleep, and low stress, you will find youth more attainable than you ever imagined.

THE ROAD TO PHYSICAL HEALTH

Physical health is the foundation of WHealth, and lifestyle modification in the form of exercise, counting calories, sleeping well, and reducing stress drives substantial reductions in the prevalence of disease and premature death.

I don't want you to take my word for this. I invite you to join me and enjoy the evidence presented in seven major research milestones we have celebrated since the turn of the century.[40, 41, 42, 43, 44, 45, 46] There is no question today that lifestyle modification has profound value in delivering WHealth!

SEVEN MAJOR RESEARCH STUDIES PROVE THAT LIFESTYLE MODIFICATION UNLOCKS PHYSICAL HEALTH

YEAR	STUDY	CONCLUSION
2001	Nurses Health Study	92% Reduction in Type 2 Diabetes
2004	INTERHEART Study Group	90% Reduction in Heart Attack
2006	Health Professionals Study	62% Reduction in Heart Disease
2007	Swedish Mammography Cohort	77% Reduction in Heart Attack
2008	Health Professionals Study & Nurses Health Study	50% Reduction in Stroke
2014	MORGEN Study	83% Reduction in Cardiovascular Disease
2014	Swedish Men's Study	79% Reduction in Heart Attack

LIFESTYLE MODIFICATION IS REWARDED WITH SIGNIFICANT REDUCTION IN RISK OF COMMON DISEASES

Heart attack, heart disease, stroke, and diabetes are all dramatically reduced through weight control, a healthy diet, moderate exercise, modest alcool consumption, and the elimination of smoking.

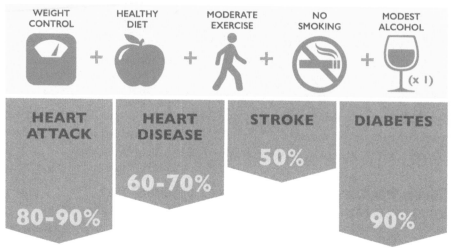

FROM NURSES HEALTH STUDY, INTERHEART STUDY GROUP, AND HEALTH PROFESSIONALS STUDY

QUALITY SLEEP HAS REAL IMPACT ON HEALTH

A good night's sleep substantially reduces the risk of fatal cardiovascular disease by a significant 16 percent, *over and above* the benefit driven by other lifestyle interventions.

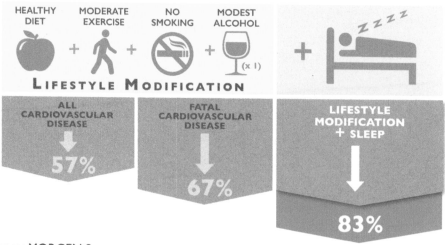

FROM MORGEN STUDY

16% ADDITIONAL RISK REDUCTION

STRESS REDUCTION DRIVES ADDITIONAL BENEFIT

Stress robs us of WHealth, and stress control drives incremental risk reduction *over and above* traditional lifestyle interventions.

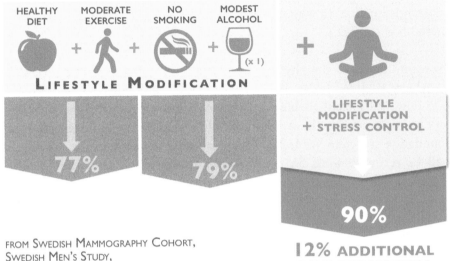

HEALTHY DIET + MODERATE EXERCISE + NO SMOKING + MODEST ALCOHOL (x 1)

LIFESTYLE MODIFICATION

+

LIFESTYLE MODIFICATION + STRESS CONTROL

77%

79%

90%

FROM SWEDISH MAMMOGRAPHY COHORT, SWEDISH MEN'S STUDY, AND INTERHEART STUDY GROUP

12% ADDITIONAL RISK REDUCTION

CONCLUSION

Your body moves by default toward decay. Through your life, the forces of degeneration overcome the forces of rejuvenation, with two major consequences: disease, and accelerated aging. Both increase your risk of premature death and, more importantly, compromise the quality of your life!

Inflammation plays a critical role in decay. Systemic inflammatory overload impacts your biological clock at the genetic level and is implicated in many of the prevalent diseases we fear in the developed world: heart disease, stroke, diabetes, dementia, and cancer.

We are victims of a massive (R)evolutionary Gap. The pace of social and technological development has dramatically outstripped our biological evolution, leaving us vulnerable to the sinister ravages of inflammatory overload.

While we look forward to even deeper insight from ongoing research, the current evidence is compelling: regular exercise and weight control emphatically oppose the forces of decay, driving rejuvenation and health. In addition, good sleep contributes to a healthy, restorative anti-inflammatory balance, and augments the good work you do through exercise and weight control. On the other hand, the ravages of stress (or more appropriately, distress) are significant, impacting our metabolic and immune health substantially; that is why controlling stress through breathing or other methods is so vital.

Now you know all the physical modifications you need to make in order to achieve BodyWHealth. In the next section of the book, we will explore two powerful mental enablers of BodyWHealth; together, these will help you to implement the lifestyle modifications required to build the physical foundation for your WHealth. Once you have established this base, you will be ready to work on emotional WHealth, the grand prize on the BodyWHealth journey.

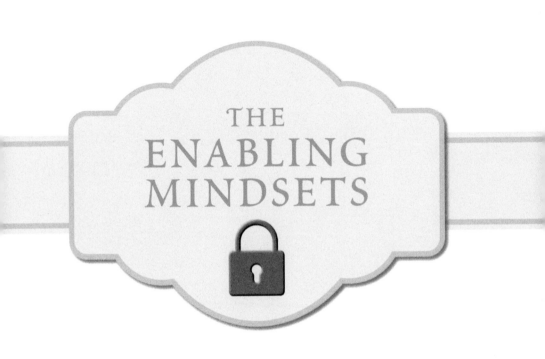

THE
ENABLING
MINDSETS

The Enabling Mindsets are powerful tools to accelerate your journey. They help you to manifest the discipline, faith, and inspiration required to unlock WHealth from within.

I have transformed my own life. I have walked the path of BodyWHealth and have sampled abundance. I sincerely wish the same for you. I have chosen to be very direct in describing the pathway because I think it is the best way to guide you. And the truth is that while the directions are simple, the journey is not always easy. It took me twenty-five years, and several failed attempts, before I tasted WHealth. If you listen to your friends and colleagues, you will know that many others have yet to get there. For sure, the journey is not always easy.

At times, the BodyWHealth journey may sound like it's a smooth, continuous ride from the moment of inspiration to the ecstasy of WHealth. Certainly the first three Keys might make it appear that way. That would be glorious, and this book would be a fairy tale. I'd love to write a fairy tale. Even more, I'd love to live one!

But like any other journey, your journey to WHealth will include ups and downs, easy runs and slow walks. It is possible you may intermittently lose your way, or occasionally forget your ultimate destination. It is likely that you will find yourself sliding backward at times, the end point receding in front of you, your past rapidly approaching from behind. That's normal.

No, BodyWHealth is not a fairy tale. It's better than that. It's the story of a hero's journey—*your* journey.

Once you have tasted WHealth, you will be hooked. Even if the roller coaster of life takes over again, and you slip back into old patterns, you will have the mental image and the taste of WHealth in your memory. Retracing your steps will be so much easier, because you appreciate the downstream reward, especially once you have developed the enabling mindsets I'm going to describe.

This section of the book describes two Keys that will enable you to implement the first three Keys to WHealth much more effectively. You will learn that excuses permit failure. You will learn that your brain can be programmed for success: first, by ingraining healthy habits; and second, by embracing *belief*, an immensely powerful mindset that drives success. As with the first three

Keys, these next two Keys are substantiated by science and tested in real life. I promise, from personal experience, that they work!

Prepare to augment your commitment, determination, and skill. Your journey, for now, remains focused on your Body, even as your eyes probe the horizon for the first signs of WHealth. Be patient; it will be yours.

KEY #4: CONQUER EXCUSES

Make a commitment that leaves no space for excuses.

George Washington Carver was a scientist and inventor born into slavery in the mid-1800s in Missouri. He spent his life working for both literal and intellectual freedom. He reportedly warned that 99 percent of failures are a result of people making excuses. He fought immense odds, yet recognized that success was in his own hands. No excuses.

I was a young physician during the emergence of the anti-tobacco era. Many of my colleagues refused to see smokers, claiming that as long as they smoked, they clearly hadn't made a commitment to good health. Although I didn't subscribe to this policy, I understood their position. They recognized the critical role that an unambiguous statement of commitment makes to success—the kind of commitment that says, "no excuses."

Many years later, I was living a life of good intention and poor results. I knew what I wanted to do. I knew how to do it. But I was still fifty pounds overweight and couldn't climb the stairs out of the New York subway without collapsing from exhaustion. When it came to taking action, there was always an excuse. Too cold. Too tired. Jet-lagged. Too many work obligations. All valid *explanations*, certainly, but not valid excuses. As excuses, they were literally killing me! The day I decided to have no more excuses in my life, I took my first steps toward BodyWHealth. I'm younger at fifty than I was at forty, and I plan to continue this trend for the rest of my life.

As a boy, I envied my friends who had those little military figurines with short, cropped hair and exquisite, manly physiques. Later, they were my own sons' favorite toys: GI Joe in the USA, Action Man in our native South Africa, and I'm sure they go by different names all around the world. I used to admire and envy their chiseled shapes, their bulging muscles, and their macho six-packs. For many years, in the back of my mind, I aspired to one day look like these fictional heroes. People like those figurines exist in real life. We all know at least one, and I still admire them today.

As I traveled my life path, I began to realize what it took to get that chiseled physique—it required an absolutely relentless, ruthless commitment to the physical self. I think I "grew up" the day I realized that this wasn't me, and it wasn't ever going to be the vast majority of the population either, because we have other opposing character traits (like lenience, sensitivity, and compromise), all of which are fundamentally good. We are never going to be chiseled works of steel that can be centerpieces of military history museums. That's okay.

So, as I urge you today to say "no excuses" for yourself, I'm not proposing this relentless, machine-like self-discipline. But I am telling you that you absolutely need to adopt a "no excuses" policy when it comes to the Keys to WHealth. Otherwise, there is no way to achieve BodyWHealth. It's that simple!

Demanding no excuses might sound like a negative thing, and BodyWHealth is predominantly a positive journey. The reason I ask for no excuses anyway is that I believe deep in my heart, after watching others and experiencing a personal transformation, that you will not achieve BodyWHealth if you allow excuses to erode your commitment. I started my personal transformation in the middle of winter. Had I allowed the snow and ice to stop my exercise, I would not be where I am today: fifty pounds lighter and several years younger than when I started. Go for it. No excuses.

For WHealth Seekers, part of not making excuses is finding ways to motivate themselves beyond the need for them. Start by writing down your BodyWHealth commitment, in simple terms. Write something like, *Today I commit myself to #1 building toward 10,000 steps, and to #2 counting calories every day for seven weeks, and to #3 sleeping better; no excuses.* Then read what you wrote out loud. Share it with your close friends. Proclaim your intention to the world. The acts of declaring and sharing are immensely powerful forces. BodyWHealth is within your grasp. Declare it to the world, eliminate excuses, and you'll find a lot of fans to support you on your journey.

Luckily, you can enlist a special natural force to help you with your "no excuse" policy. Recurring behavior becomes etched into your brain as *habit.* The mechanical act of repetition is an immensely powerful motivator and can drive you toward the negative ("you're in a rut") or the positive ("you're in the zone"). Positive, motivating habit is born when WHealth Seekers embrace and live the "no excuses" mindset.

Whether you're starting your journey for the first time (or only just beginning to think about it), or have had a taste of BodyWHealth and slipped backward, or already have BodyWHealth and seek more, I hope that this book will inspire and support you to make no excuses on your journey. In each of these situations, you need to effect a meaningful change in your current trajectory. You need to grasp control of the steering wheel, and make bold changes to your direction or speed—without excuses. This mindset is about that change.

YOUR PRESCRIPTION FOR WHEALTH

I have fantasized about it often. "Please come in, Mrs. Nelson, have a seat. So, you'd like a new life? You want to transform? You want to feel good, every day? I can help you. We're going to change your habits, the daily actions and behaviors that drive you automatically. It won't hurt a bit. I'm going to write a prescription for you. You don't need to come back to see me for a follow-up—I know this prescription will work!"

Each time I woke from this fantasy, I found a real person sitting in my consulting room, someone I really wanted to help. Unfortunately, a simple prescription, a little piece of paper with a few scribbled words, wasn't useful. I needed more than that to help my patients profoundly change their lives. I needed BodyWHealth, a systematic, disciplined way to inspire WHealthy actions.

You're now sitting with me, reading this book. I believe it is possible to transform your life, particularly with science as your friend.

The destination is WHealth, but that is not our immediate focus. You will achieve WHealth by working on your daily actions and behaviors, your habits. You don't drive from New York City to San Diego by dreaming of life at the Pacific Ocean. You get into your car, fill it with gas, punch an address into your GPS, and then press the accelerator and brake pedal a million times. That's how you have to achieve BodyWHealth, too. The journey is the actions: pushing on the accelerator and brake pedal a million times, almost without thinking about it. You need to be able to exercise, balance calories, and sleep well in this same automated, habitual fashion on your way to WHealth.

So how do you automate your life, embracing new, WHealthy actions and behaviors in an enduring manner? Through the fourth Key to WHealth: *Make a commitment that leaves no space for excuses.* In order to accomplish this, I recommend an approach I call the *Rule of Sevens*—breaking the process up into seven days, seven weeks, and seven months, because those are the critical time intervals that social scientists and biologists have identified on the journey to meaningful change.

The essence of this approach is to set a few milestones to work toward, and then to reward yourself handsomely when you get to them. In doing so, you break down the journey into manageable bites. It is demotivating to contemplate the end goal while you're laboring through the early steps. Using sevens, you can set yourself short-term goals that are within your grasp. You can co-opt the enormous power of affirmation to fuel your journey. If you stick to the program, after an almost poetic nine months (the sum of seven days, seven weeks, and seven months), you will have the taste of BodyWHealth. It will be hard to turn back from there.

The first seven days are critical to breaking the inertia of your old way of life. It's like beginning a road trip; starting your car's engine is more work than keeping it going. These are crucial days because good intentions wane quickly. If you started your 10,000 steps with a walk around the block (that's a great start, by the way!), you may find yourself saying, "Well, I'm so far from my goal, and it's cold in the mornings now, so I'm going to skip tomorrow"… and the day after you do the same…and then you're beat. You could argue that the greatest gains are made by early repetition, so devote yourself with singular resolve to the first seven days. For subsequent periods of time, the chemicals in your brain will begin to help to reinforce your motivation, but those first seven days take plain and simple *willpower*. Take your steps, count your calories, and sleep well with devotion for seven days, not skipping a single day, no excuses! After seven days, you will have affirmed you positive intent and desire for change.

Then, reward yourself. Use something small. Something meaningful. Something that puts a smile on your face for the full next week and inspires you to continue stepping out and counting calories and sleeping well without skipping a single day. You *must* reward yourself. Don't say, "Oh, that was easy; I'll save the reward for another day." Even though you understand that you're playing a game with yourself, the immediate reward is still important. The pleasure of your achievement plus the pleasure of the reward combine to release powerful chemicals in your brain that will help you on the next stage of your journey.

That next stage of your journey is setting your sights on the milestone of seven weeks. Why seven weeks? Because studies show that the vast majority of people become entrenched in a new habit within forty-two days (six weeks); I add an extra week just to make sure. It is a beautiful number, and during those seven weeks, some crucial chemical and behavioral adaptations will be taking place in your body. Your objective is to implement the first three Keys fully, each week, for the duration. Once you have practiced your good behaviors for seven weeks, you're well on your way to fundamental life change—to WHealth!

Successfully completing those seven weeks calls for a really big celebration, something that you will remember for a long time. Don't be thrifty. Choose something that you wouldn't ordinarily do, something that stretches the envelope. You're making the most important change in your life. You're on your way to BodyWHealth, a destination of abundant WHealth. These seven weeks are simple, but not easy, and you've done it! Again, you must reward yourself. For seven weeks your brain has craved the rewarding chemicals you tempted it with at the seven-day milestone. Reward it, and it will work for you again on the next part of the journey.

By now, you can guess what's coming. You are going to plan the mother and father of all celebrations, a reward that will stand out in your mind as a powerful beacon as you continue your commitment—without excuses—for the next seven months. During that time, your objective is to continue walking 10,000 steps on at least five days of each week, counting calories every day, and sleeping enough every night. In truth, by the end of seven months, you will probably be quite good at estimating your daily energy intake and burn, and you will probably be pretty close to your desired weight. Hopefully, you will be sleeping long and well, and controlling your stress better, too—and you might even be working toward the emotional mastery we will explore in the next section of this book. But to earn your reward, you need to be able to look yourself in your eyes in the mirror, knowing that you have consistently met your exercise, energy, and sleep goals for the full seven-month duration—no excuses. If you can maintain the discipline and enthusiasm to meet this goal, then you will understand how to transform your life. You will have laid the tracks for enduring lifestyle modification. You will have set the physical foundation for BodyWHealth. Enjoy the prize!

THE SCIENCE OF SEVENS

To appreciate the Rule of Sevens, we need to understand the science that underlies habit. Not surprisingly, this is all controlled in our nerve center, the brain. It is not controlled at the cortical level (the gray matter that helps us to think and reason), but much deeper, in areas known as the *brain stem* and *dorsal ganglia*. Here we find primitive circuits that regulate cravings. Two chemical systems are involved. The *dopamine system* evokes desire and motivation. It drives seeking and searching behavior. The other system is the *opioid system*. It evokes sensations of pleasure. To attain BodyWHealth, we want to activate dopamine desire circuits as well as the opioid reward system in a way that impels us to recurrent, automated WHealthy behavior (or habits).

You may have heard about *endorphins*. They are natural opioid chemicals that are produced after exercise and makes us feel really, really good! But we don't start craving them after our first bout of exercise. It takes a little while. The discipline of forcing ourselves to exercise for seven days, then for seven weeks, then for seven months allows our body to make the chemical changes necessary to activate this chemical reward system.

This is not only true for exercise. Scientists believe there are similar changes happening for other habits, too—both good and bad habits. During the early period of habit-forming, chemical sensitization and rewiring happens. The result is that as you progress, your dependence on willpower declines, and your body's natural craving-reward cycle takes over. For WHealth Seekers like you, that means that by about seven weeks, you will have engaged your physiological autopilot toward the BodyWHealth destination!

Similarly, through psychosocial research into habit and behavioral change, we have identified a three-step, self-reinforcing cycle that can be either virtuous (good habits) or destructive (bad habits). The first step in the habit cycle is the activation of a *trigger* or *cue*. It precipitates the *routine*, or habitual behavior we are interested in establishing (the second step). Finally, the routine is *rewarded* in the third step.

Here is an example of this cycle at work: Mr. Nelson arrives home at the end of his workday (trigger). He walks to the kitchen, opens the refrigerator, and cracks open a beer (routine). He puts his feet up and relaxes as the alcohol calms him down (reward). Does this scene sound familiar?

Now imagine how we can turn this bad habit into a WHealthy habit, using the same underlying science…

Mr. Nelson arrives home at the end of his workday (same trigger). He greets his wife and walks to the bedroom to put on his exercise clothes (new routine). He adds 7,000 steps to the 3,000 he already achieved at work, flooding his blood with endorphins that make him relax and feel good (new, but similar, reward).

That's the trick and the purpose for the Rule of Sevens! You use your willpower to boost yourself to the point where your body has installed new circuitry, and habit takes over from there. It's beautiful!

DOPAMINE AND OPIOID SYSTEMS FUEL RECURRENT, AUTOMATED BEHAVIOR, OR HABIT

Deep within your brain, in the brain stem and dorsal ganglia, primitive neural circuits and chemicals regulate cravings.

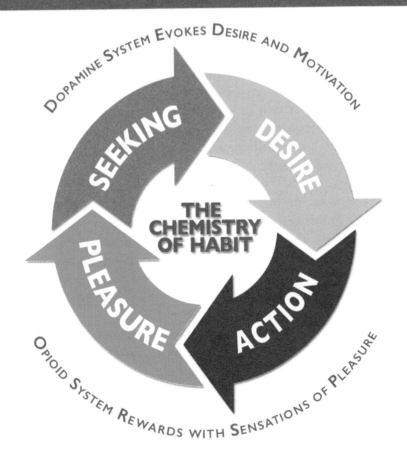

SIMPLE RECOMMENDATIONS FOR CONQUERING EXCUSES

1. *Build a hierarchy of reward.* One of my favorite WHealth Seekers pasted pictures of her rewards onto a wall calendar. At seven days, she pasted a picture of the most beautiful red evening gown—one she had been admiring for some time, but couldn't justify buying. Now she had earned it! At seven weeks, she posted a picture of a limousine driving up to a luxurious hotel. This image motivated her to move it and count calories, and after seven weeks, her husband opened the door of that limo to allow her to step out with her new body and blossoming confidence on their way to a weekend of pampered luxury. Finally, the photo of the exotic island retreat she pasted at seven months into her journey motivated her toward that life-changing milestone. These images celebrated her new life of enduring WHealth. Don't be shy when you choose your rewards. They will help you to a new life of inestimable value.

2. *Chart your progress.* Jerry Seinfeld boasted a productivity tracker that helped him to be disciplined about his creative writing. He pinned a calendar on his wall and placed a big red X onto each day that he wrote his comedy. After a few days, he had a chain of big red X's, like little people holding hands across his wall. His driving obsession became not to break the chain. You can copy Seinfeld's approach with your own wall or desk calendar, or even an electronic version. There are mobile phone apps that harness this principle. You can record "winning streaks" (the number of days you go without breaking the chain) and tap into your competitive side to make it more fun!

3. *Put it out there.* The internal commitment that comes from an external statement of that commitment is a powerful force for enduring change. Write your intentions down. Don't capture them as just a wish or desire, but as a positive statement, a fact. Tell your friends and family. Saying your goals out loud reinforces your intentions, and earns you some fans on the sidelines to cheer you on. Embrace their scrutiny and support.

4. *Buddy up.* For some strange reason, we all believe our own excuses more than others do. So when I pull back the curtain and say, "It's cold this morning; I think I'll sleep in for another thirty minutes," it seems very reasonable to me. To my exercise partner who is already standing outside next to my mailbox, it sounds really lame!

5. ***Understand and break the cycle of shame.*** We all feel bad when we offer up an excuse. First, we feel bad for not delivering on a promise. Then we feel bad because we've dredged up a reason for not delivering—and most of the time, in our heart of hearts, we know that our explanation is weak. There is huge risk in this cycle of shame because it becomes self-reinforcing. We begin by *feeling* bad, and we end up believing we *are* bad. If you stumble on your journey of good intentions, be very careful about the words you use in your head. There is a profound difference between saying "I am bad" and saying "I did something bad." If you miss your steps goal for a week, don't beat yourself up. Just know that you'll try again the next week. It also helps when you catch yourself feeling guilty to replace that guilt very quickly with gratitude. As you hear yourself saying, "I feel bad because I didn't walk today," stop! Then force the following sentence into your mind: "I am grateful that I have good strong legs, and I am excited to walk again tomorrow!" Gratitude is a powerful force!

6. ***Find inspirational quotes and pictures.*** Gifted writers and speakers are able to package tons of energy into a few carefully crafted words or sentences. Photographs and pictures can reach deep into your soul to touch and inspire your own creative forces. Put them up on the wall, on sticky notes on your desk or refrigerator, on your calendar, or in your sneakers. There are also an expanding number of apps that will send you a daily motivator. These will help you avoid the temptation to make excuses.

7. ***Play games.*** Games are fun, provide incentive, and reinforce habit. Many employers and big corporations are starting to deploy fun health-promoting games into their formerly gray benefit packages. There are several health apps available to appeal to your competitive instincts, allowing you to compete with friends and family in healthy activities. I see many 10,000-step games where you can encourage friends, family, and coworkers toward their health goals, even as you stride forward on your own WHealth journey.

8. ***Know when it's okay to make an excuse.*** I know I keep emphasizing the "no excuses" concept, and that's generally a good rule to follow. But there are certain circumstances—for example, if you are ill, or a doctor has told you to restrict motion—under which it may be appropriate for you to pause your BodyWhealth behavior, such as exercise, momentarily. Just remember to jump back into your WHealthy habits as soon as you can!

CONCLUSION

Beginning the journey to WHealth may be simple, but it isn't easy. You will probably be very tempted to make excuses along the way. But if you can dig deep into your stores of willpower and push past those early wobbly moments, motivating yourself through rewards until those rewards entrench your habit, you will soon find that you have formed WHealthy habits that will carry you through seven days, then seven weeks, then seven months, until you can't imagine why you would have made an excuse in the first place.

WHealth Plus

In addition to making no excuses and rewarding yourself for achieving seven days, seven weeks, and seven months of WHealthy behaviors, I advocate that you make celebration a regular part of your BodyWHealth journey. While it is important that milestone celebrations stand out above others, the emotional and physical reward of ongoing celebration should be a pervasive part of WHealth. Two components of celebration are particularly valuable: Gratitude and affirmation are both powerful forces that unlock WHealth.

THE POWER OF GRATITUDE: APPRECIATION DRIVES HAPPINESS

Do you want ten minutes of happiness? Sit quietly with a pen and paper and write down all the ways you can say "thank you." Remember how people have thanked you in the past, and how you have thanked them. Remember everything about the experience: the sight, sound, touch, smell, and (if appropriate) taste. I guarantee you very happy memories and a profoundly uplifting experience.

Gratitude is the outward expression of a deeply powerful inner emotion, *appreciation.* This profoundly positive state generates a physiological and psychological environment in which we thrive both physically and emotionally. This is BodyWHealth!

Gratitude, a continuous state of thankfulness, has been shown to impact our health in very real ways. Studies have demonstrated that it can reduce our blood pressure, easing the burden that high blood pressure puts on our hearts. Gratitude also increases the presence of beneficial immune cells and other chemicals that equip us to better ward off cancer and infection. Gratitude's link with long-term emotional health is convincing, and happiness has a strong positive impact on both immune health and longevity.

We know that many of the associated phenomena that accompany appreciation, like love, empathy, smiling, and laughter, all have proven health benefits. Reaching out to others is equally powerful, both in the physical sense where touch is a strong stimulant of health and in the emotional sense where generosity and kindness benefit the giver.

When we express our appreciation toward others by showing gratitude, we complete a virtuous loop. By strengthening any stage in the loop, social scientists believe that we can reinforce the overall impact of the cycle. When we express gratitude, we invoke our brain in an almost automated fashion, bringing happiness and reward into our own lives, elevating our mood and spirits. In turn, we say "thanks" more often and more meaningfully. In addition to the good we do in the world, the personal payback is immense. You express gratitude, then feel good, then express more gratitude…and so on, and so on, moving you invariably toward health and happiness.

Say thank you, often. Find new ways to express your gratitude, and keep a gratitude diary. You can do this simply by writing a gratitude statement on top of each page in your daily planner. You could buy a glamorous journal and script beautiful prose using your advanced calligraphy skills to make this a visual pleasure ground. There are numerous electronic tools that can help, too, and several highly attractive apps for mobile phones. You can include photographs and add social context by linking with friends. You can use your social media pages to chronicle your appreciation in a very personal way. However you choose to approach this, don't forget the fundamentals: to simply say "thank you" both authentically and frequently. This is a powerful tool to drive both emotional and physical WHealth!

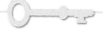

"Gratitude is not only the greatest of virtues,
but the parent of all others."

CICERO

THE POWER OF AFFIRMATION:
GOOD FOR YOU AND GOOD FOR OTHERS

I have a treasured book that occupies a very special place on my bookshelf. The book is *Whale Done*, and the principal authors are leadership guru Ken Blanchard and Jim Ballard. Their coauthors Thad Lacinak and Chuck Thompkins are marine mammal trainers from Sea World. The gentle beauty of this story lies in the underlying knowledge that marine mammals like dolphins only respond to positive reinforcement.

You can train a dolphin to dive deep below the surface of a pool, circle three times in opposite directions from its mates, then leap high into the air to do a front flip before tipping a ball with its nose…but only by rewarding it. Negative feedback, criticism, and punishment have no place in dolphin training. In fact, as with human beings, these destructive tactics are counterproductive, making the beautiful, sensitive animals insecure and unwilling to cooperate with their human trainers.

Instead, empathetic trainers employ the immense power of affirmation and reward their animal students liberally for success. In the beginning, they work hard to "catch" a young mammal doing the "right" things. A combination of kind words, warm tactile rewards in the form of pats and rubs, and fishy treats affirm the actions of the animal. This affirmation triggers a flood of pleasurable chemical sensations in its brain, at once rewarding it for its actions and incenting it toward additional learning.

Imagine how impactful we would be in our own lives if we could master the power of affirmation. Self-affirmation is a valuable self-training tool. Enlisting others in your celebration makes it even more powerful. A positive word from a spouse, partner, child, or parent in a moment of spontaneous celebration is dynamite. And the beauty is that affirming others is itself an act of generosity with its own health benefits. So when your spouse, partner, child, or parent affirms you, they are also giving themselves a WHealthy boost. It is a wonderful cycle that perpetuates WHealth for everyone involved.

Explore the power of affirmation to *celebrate* BodyWHealth, reinforcing forever WHealthy habits in you and your loved ones!

Congratulations on your exceptional progress! You have learned—and are hopefully using—four of the seven Keys to WHealth. You are now ready for the biggest insight I've discovered about BodyWHealth. It is the most powerful tool for unlocking health, happiness, and prosperity. This will be the most exciting part of your journey. Please join me in the next chapter to explore this life-altering mindset, the most powerful Key to WHealth.

KEY #5: BELIEVE

Believe to achieve.

Here is the greatest lesson of all: the single most powerful action to unlocking WHealth. The fifth Key has far-reaching implications well beyond your health and happiness. It taps into a life force you can command, as well as skills you can learn and practice that will change your life in any domain you choose. It is *the* Key that will transform your desire for health and happiness into enduring, life-changing WHealth.

THE POWER TO CHANGE LIVES: **BELIEVE**

I quit my job and moved to San Diego to write this book. The day I told somebody in my new hometown that I was an author, the book started taking shape. Something changed deep inside my brain the moment I began to believe in myself as an author. Interestingly, a similar quantum leap started my personal journey to BodyWHealth.

I was over halfway through my forties, a physician and exercise scientist. I had seen the consequences of physical neglect in my clinical practice and research. I understood the science intimately. Yet there I was, fifty pounds overweight, unable to walk up a long flight of stairs without resting. With a beautiful wife and four amazing, growing children whom I loved dearly, I had every reason to want to stay healthy for a long time. I understood the first four Keys to WHealth—to exercise, to count calories, to sleep well, and to work unrelentingly at good, excuse-free habits. Nevertheless, I was stuck in that very bad place, unable to put those principles into action.

The fifth Key is arguably the most powerful and most important of the seven navigational beacons for BodyWHealth. It transformed my good intentions into sustained healthy behavior. More than that, it gave me reason to believe that there is WHealth beyond health. It keeps me motivated and working hard even now that I am WHealthy, because there are no limits to WHealth.

What I'm proposing may sound trite at first: *Believe to achieve*. When I began my journey to WHealth, I thought I believed, and I did…intellectually. I knew that exercise induces chemical and structural changes in the body that are rewarded by health and happiness. Despite this, I remained stuck in the same world of bad habits that had colored the last decade of my life.

Then suddenly one day, almost by accident, I looked in the mirror and saw a young man and an athlete. That single moment changed everything. I vividly remember every detail of that transformative experience. Sure, I saw the same reflection I had seen the day before: the same bulges and sags that arise with neglect and middle age. But I didn't stop in that negative, superficial image. I looked through the façade and *believed* that the man behind it was young, fit, and healthy. And then, miraculously, I was! Because I believed I was an athlete, I acted like one. I exercised like an athlete (starting slowly, of course). I ate like an athlete, skipping the extra donut. I slept like an athlete. I made no excuses, not because I had exceptional willpower, but because a real athlete simply wouldn't. I pictured, *believed*, and then lived that future. Three years later, I had lost fifty pounds, could run up a flight of steps without pausing, and more. I was five years younger than when I started and had tasted prosperity, in its broadest sense.

I strongly urge you to reread the previous paragraph. It captures the most powerful lesson I could ever teach a WHealth Seeker. I will substantiate my experience with the underlying science, and you will see numerous quotes in this chapter from people who are way more famous than I am, and who understand the profound force of this insight. But the simple description of what actually happened in my own brain, and then my own life, remains the most convincing evidence I can muster. My greatest wish for you is that you have a similar experience to the one I had. It will transform you, forever.

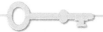

*"The only person you are destined to become
is the person you decide to be."*

RALPH WALDO EMERSON

The good news is that I had earned that moment—which means you can earn your own moment, too. I had worked earnestly to find the secret to sustained behavioral change. Then suddenly, standing in front of the mirror of my wife's dressing table, my efforts were rewarded.

There are many verbs that spring into action as soon as you *believe*. Once you believe that you are fit, healthy, and athletic, you start *planning, intending, anticipating, expecting, attracting, manifesting,* and *trusting* the behavior required to drive WHealth. For many years, I taught elite athletes to visualize themselves competing in and winning their specific event in order to deliver the very success they dreamt about. I constantly advise patients, clients, work colleagues, and my own children to believe that we have within our own hearts and minds the ability to affect our destiny. Despite teaching this truth for many years, I had never experienced it with such power until my own revolutionizing moment. In an instant, my life was transformed.

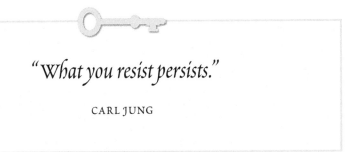

"What you resist persists."

CARL JUNG

So what does this mean for your WHealth? And how would I go about this transformation again, perhaps in another domain of my life?

The first part is to start by focusing on what you have, and being grateful for it. Say it out loud, or write it down. "I am thankful for the two strong legs that will help me walk. I am grateful that I have a beautiful wife and four amazing children, and the will to be with them as they grow up. I appreciate that I still have time to make a difference in my own life, and to achieve WHealth." Out of gratefulness comes resolve.

The second part is to focus on what you want, and *not* on what you *don't* want. This is necessary because belief works both ways. This is a subtle but immensely powerful concept. Sometimes, we spend more mental energy looking at the bars of the prison we are trying to escape from than we do contemplating either the reward or the act of escaping. This becomes self-defeating. You have to spend more time thinking about the slim, healthy person you are (or will be) than the unhealthy, unattractive person you are accustomed to seeing in the mirror. If you spend your time bemoaning or resisting being overweight, your mind remains occupied with negative images, you continually reinforce the belief that you are overweight, and guess what? It persists, and you remain overweight.

The opposite of belief is *fear* or *doubt*. In the case of health, *shame* and *embarrassment* are also powerful enemies. They appear, working to erode your belief in the new you, when you look in the mirror or stand on your bathroom scale. That is why I talk about weight sparingly (focusing instead on calories and energy balance) and will seldom advocate that you use your bathroom scale. In fact, I hope that you remember that I suggest getting rid of your bathroom scale entirely, because when you stand on it, you will spend more time thinking about being overweight than being the slim, healthy person you want to be.

In the beginning, belief is very difficult. It's hard to see and believe in the new you. Doubt intervenes pretty quickly; you argue with yourself and relapse to seeing yourself with old eyes. On another level, knowledge of the power of belief can be frightening. It's easier to blame somebody else or something else for what is wrong. In truth, each one of us has the power to see and deliver BodyWHealth to ourselves, and that's both exhilarating and liberating.

Now let me be clear. I'm not advocating for a blind belief that anything is possible. We all have physical limits to our biological elasticity. We're not all going to be Olympic athletes. Certain biological changes are beyond our mental control. We still need physicians, and we might still need medicine. I still take my cholesterol medication every day. What I profoundly believe is that each and every one of us can always achieve more. Regardless of your physical condition, BodyWHealth is attainable. It's the best investment you can make.

In the early stages of developing belief, it's easier to find things to be grateful for than to believe, and as with many things, practice improves your skill. So keep up the gratitude as a daily ritual, because it will ultimately help you believe. Affirmation is the most powerful psychological driver, whether coming from self or from others. You'll remember from the fourth Key that reward entrenches good habits. When you celebrate your BodyWHealth, you reinforce healthy behavior, declare future intentions (*believe*), and—via a host of hormones and neurotransmitters (chemicals in the brain that we will discuss in depth later in this chapter)—entrench a voracious appetite for more success!

> *"The only thing that stands between you and your dream is the will to try and the belief that it is actually possible."*
>
> JOEL BROWN

WORDS OF THE WISE, THE SUCCESSFUL, AND THE WHEALTHY

Nelson Mandela is my hero. Above all other mortals, he captures for me the vision, courage, determination, fortitude, love, and forgiveness of a great leader. He worked against incredible odds, and succeeded. In fact, he went beyond success. His aura and work eclipsed the massive challenge he took on, to overthrow the evil of apartheid and its formal constitutional construct. His example inspires great leaders from every corner of the globe, and simple folk like you and me. Through twenty-seven crushing years in prison, he *believed*. He *believed* in his vision. He *believed* in his rights. He *believed* that he would liberate the people of South Africa. He *believed* that he would lead us to freedom. And he did!

Through his long years of incarceration, Madiba (the familiar name we use for Mandela, denoting great respect and love for the man and his family) held a Victorian poem close to his heart. The poem, entitled "Invictus" (which means "unconquered"), was written by William Ernest Henley a century before Madiba was thrown into the apartheid dungeons on the infamous Robben Island. Not surprisingly, the concluding lines of this great masterpiece reflect not only Madiba's inextinguishable belief, but also the unshakeable knowledge that his future was firmly *in his own hands*.

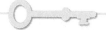

"I am the master of my fate; I am the captain of my soul."

In August 1963, Martin Luther King, Jr., revealed the same power of *belief* when he shared his "I have a dream" speech with over 250,000 civil rights supporters on the steps of the Lincoln Memorial. Although he uses the somewhat gentler imagery of a "dream," his steely conviction and *belief* resound throughout his passionate description of the future he sees. Few can dispute that the power of this great leader's belief has resulted in dramatic, sweeping changes in the United States.

Why my obsession with successful people? We all know somebody who has the power to make a difference. Nelson Mandela, Martin Luther King, Jr., and Mahatma Gandhi are my icons. Each of you will have your own heroes, great leaders who have achieved success across a wide range of life. Think Steve Jobs, Winston Churchill, the Pope, Indira Gandhi, the Dalai Lama, Teddy Roosevelt, Eleanor Roosevelt, Albert Einstein, Princess Diana, Rosa Parks, and Mother Teresa. We can learn from them to help us achieve BodyWHealth. They share a common power that elevates them above others. We would probably each call it something different—confidence, determination, intention—but at the core, what they share is *belief*.

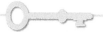

"Whether you think you can,
or think you can't—you're right."

HENRY FORD

The name we give it doesn't really matter. I choose the word "belief" because it describes for me the deep faith in a current or future state that compels appropriate action and makes success inevitable. I also choose the word "belief" because it accurately reflects the neuroscience that underpins this power. Henry Ford recognized this, too, when he identified the role our thoughts play in our future. Thoughts originate somewhere in our brain. When you read on, you will discover the fascinating science that surrounds the inner battle to moderate the power of our thoughts. For now, it is enough to agree that they play a profound role in determining our future.

There is abundant evidence that regular people have enjoyed extraordinary achievements by believing in success and refusing to contemplate failure. In her book *The Secret*, Rhonda Byrne labels the power that fuels success as "intention." She goes on to describe what she calls "the Law of Attraction," which (loosely) states that you become what you think about most. I profoundly believe her message, which is supported by the strong evidence for the power of *belief* seen in modern neuroscience.

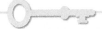

> *"Whatever you can do, or dream you can do, begin it.*
> *Boldness has genius, power, and magic in it."*
>
> GOETHE

Don't get me wrong. I don't believe that there is a magical force or state of mind that simply unlocks success without any additional effort. Hard work is still part of the equation. Change must also be consistent with reality. But *belief* is the starting point, and the fuel, and the power, and the inspiration, and the guide on the transformative journey.

We are about to embark on an exploratory journey into your brain, to understand the biology of belief. You will discover that you are able to learn and practice skills that enhance your powers of belief. These are potent tools that will help you on your BodyWHealth journey, and well beyond.

THE ANATOMY OF BELIEF

In order to understand the interrelationship between our *belief* and our brain, we need to review the evolution of this powerful organ. The current human brain reflects the incremental progress of hundreds of millions of years. Starting with a very primitive brain, Mother Nature has added faculties and capabilities in successive layers of neurological, mental, and psychosocial development. Today we enjoy the most complex and powerful brain on the planet.

LEVELS OF THE BRAIN

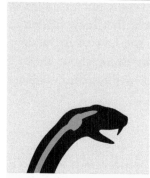

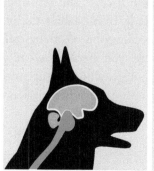

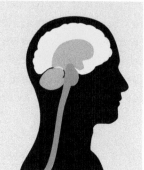

PRIMITIVE BRAIN
Controls survival urges, fight and flight responses. Fear center.

EMOTIONAL BRAIN
Source of emotions like love and empathy. Craves community interaction.

COGNITIVE BRAIN
Center of higher thought. Drives reason, logic, and abstract awareness.

At the center of our brain, in the most primitive part of our central nervous system, we supervise critical *survival* instincts. The *primitive* brain (also known as the *reptilian* brain) is responsible for fight and flight responses. It is the default brain we use in times of crisis. Driven by fear and adrenaline, this part of our brain drives us to flee from danger or turn to meet it with aggression. We need our primitive brains, but if that was all we had, we would be cold survival engines, like snakes and lizards.

Over time, early mammals added the limbic system to their primitive brains. The limbic system brought emotion and color to our world. This *emotional* brain provides a selective advantage to those species that have it, because it drives them to love and nurture their offspring, and to collaborate with others. We humans have the limbic system layered around our primitive brain stems. The language of the emotional brain is love and empathy.

Finally, we humans added a massive cerebral cortex to those first two components, increasing our brain to three times the size of our closest mammalian relatives. This *cognitive* layer in the brain introduced thought and reason to our mental resources, and clearly differentiates us from other animals. It is a powerful organ that enables us to master our environment. You will soon understand the huge importance of this power.

The three parts of our brain—primitive, emotional, and cognitive—are intimately connected. Millions of nerve junctions enable messages to pass between them, moderating their influence in our lives. Our overall behavior is the composite effect of the three brain centers. In the absence of any "higher" function, the primitive brain rules with its negative, defensive messages. "Run, hide, fight!" it screams. This is useful when we are in true danger, but it is a disruptive influence at most other times. Fortunately, both the emotional and the cognitive brains can override the primitive brain. Picture a calm and loving scene where your head is filled with empathy and passion. The furthest things from your mind are the "run, hide, fight!" messages. Your emotional brain has silenced them. Now picture a situation where you build the courage to jump from a high ledge into the deep, inviting pool of a tranquil river. Deep down, your primitive brain is shouting its defensive messages, but your cognitive brain, which has done its research and knows that it will be safe, sends quieting messages that suppress the primitive brain and enable your adventure. Some call this "mind over matter." Interestingly, we also know that the cognitive brain is able to influence our emotional brain to some extent, establishing a very distinct hierarchy among the three brain centers.

Importantly, we have varying degrees of voluntary control over the three parts of our brains. We have no direct control over the primitive brain. We know from studying people with severe brain injuries that survival reflexes persist even when higher functions are destroyed. These are powerful, autonomous reflexes. At the other end of the scale, we are maximally able to influence our cognitive brains. That's the purpose of education: to widen the exposure of our brain to different experiences and to program thought channels that enable us to more successfully activate our cerebral cortexes. The emotional brain is somewhere between the two; it has many of the features of an autonomous center, driving itself, but we can influence it indirectly via our cognitive brains, and possibly even directly (think of the effect of music on mood).

The Power of Belief

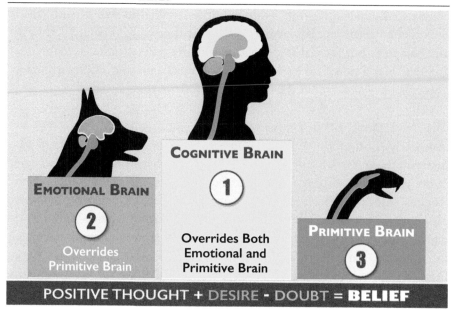

So, how do the three parts of our brain influence *belief*?

First, we start with an idea. This happens in our cognitive brains. We structure a mental image of something we *want*. We create the picture using words, or perhaps mental images. That picture alone may be enough to drive small actions. If I am thirsty and want a drink, it's not a huge deal to get up from my desk to get a glass of water. But to achieve something bigger, an idea alone is inadequate. We need to bring some emotion to the idea, to turn *want* into *desire*. That's the role of the emotional brain. To achieve something big, we need that deep, nonrational hunger for success.

But there are times when we want something huge, and even *desire* is not enough. Many of us can describe things that we truly desire. We have strong, clear ideas of them, and we also have deep emotional hungers for them. But still, I know from the statistics of life that the vast majority of these desires go unrealized. Most dreamers do not deliver success. Why?

The reason lurks in the primitive reptilian brain. Remember its function? To protect us. As we develop wants and desires, our primitive brains are doing exactly what they have been trained over millions of years to do. Even as we picture the slim, healthy body we desire, or the castle on the mountaintop, or the spectacular new job, or the freedom to travel, our primitive brains kick into action. Instead of shouting simple commands like "run, hide, fight!" they impregnate our consciousness with "protective" messages hidden in more elaborate questions. Questions like, "What happens if I fail? What will my friends and family think of me? Why should I, who have always been unsuccessful, suddenly become wealthy? Why should the world take me seriously now? Who would even listen to my concept?" Millions of brilliant ideas are thwarted every day by our powerful primitive brains.

I hope that two things are now clear to you. The first is that success is elusive, a secret understood and mastered by only a few. The second, and more important, is that for substantial success, you need to align your entire brain behind your idea. You need to evoke the power of the cognitive and emotional brains in a *desire* so powerful that it overrides all resistance that the primitive brain will invoke. This is *belief*.

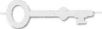

"The greatest discovery of any generation is that human beings can alter their lives by altering the attitudes of their minds."

ALBERT SCHWEITZER

THE POWER OF **BELIEF**

We have now explored the three parts of the human brain and their roles in nurturing *belief*, the most important and elusive ingredient to success. Now, we're going to explore the mental journey required to take a *desire* to grand success. You will need this to attain both BodyWHealth and every other big ambition.

The two schematics below follows a big idea from inception through to success (and the statistical projections of this model reflect real-life experience, giving

Not All Good Ideas Lead to Success

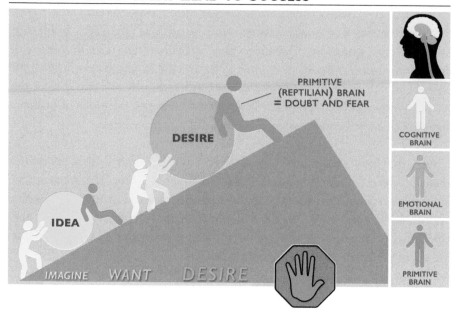

me geeky reassurance in its integrity). The bigger the idea, the more powerfully you need to evoke the pathway to *belief* in order to make it reality. Once you achieve *belief*, success is largely inevitable. If you don't believe me, study any person who has achieved grand success with a big idea. Once they *believed*, truly *believed*, plans became actions, hopes became expectations, obstacles became challenges, and success followed.

A big idea is first generated in the cognitive brain. You now *want* something. When coupled with emotion, you transform that *want* into a colorful, three-dimensional *desire*. But desire alone is not enough to overcome the retarding influence of the primitive brain that drives doubt, undermining our thoughts and hopes directly. Too many good ideas die at this stage. Even if we engage in activities to move us toward our goal, doubt sabotages our efforts. Most likely, we kill the big idea before we can achieve it. Only when the desire becomes so strong that we call it *belief* do we have the power to overcome the primitive brain and its accomplice *fear*. The result of that scenario is always success.

Several aspects of this model require further clarification. First, although we represent the process as a linear journey from left to right in the diagrams above, this is not entirely true in life. The interactions between the three levels in the brain are more iterative, more dynamic. It is not an instantaneous

BELIEF UNLOCKS SUCCESS

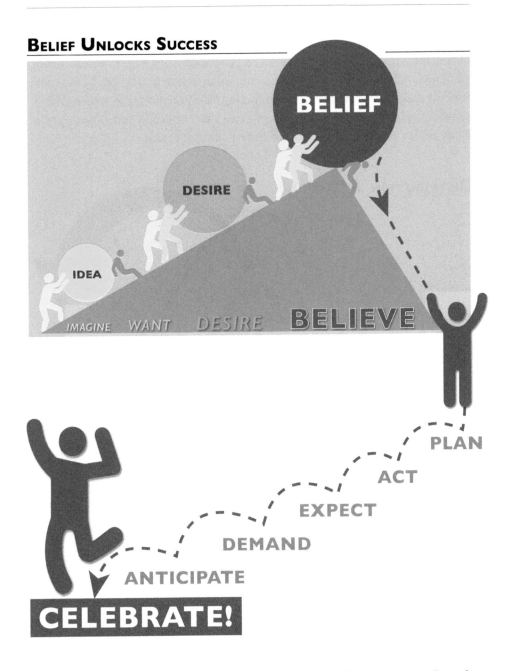

chemical reaction. Big ideas can take time to fully develop as we wrestle with our primitive brain, before we finally overcome doubt with *belief*.

Second, belief and success can be situational. We can be more proficient in developing belief in some domains of our life (perhaps our professional life), while being less confident in others (like our personal life).

Third, as you can see in the graphic below, very few people are hugely successful. Similarly, the proportion of people who are hugely unsuccessful, who never achieve *belief* at all and ultimately autodestruct, is tiny. Many more are only moderately successful at triggering *belief*, vacillating between days of enabling belief to get the upper hand and drive success, and other days of living under the defensive cloud of their primitive brains.

DISTRIBUTION OF SUCCESS

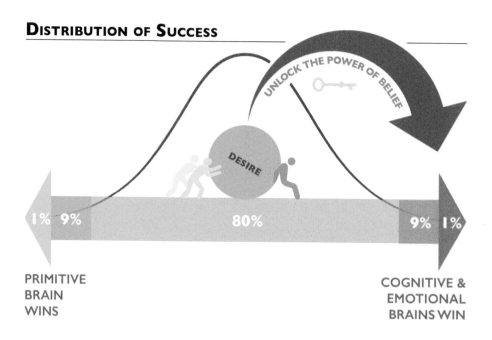

PRIMITIVE
BRAIN
WINS

COGNITIVE &
EMOTIONAL
BRAINS WIN

If we understand the roles of the three layers in our brain and the relationships between them, fully appreciate the evolutionary power of the cognitive brain, and closely observe highly successful people, we should be filled with optimism. We know that we can directly influence the cognitive brain, and we can influence the emotional brain indirectly through the cognitive brain. If we can learn to do this with sufficient strength and consistency, we can drive *belief* and enjoy success.

LIMITING BELIEFS: ROADBLOCKS TO WHEALTH

Our thoughts drive our future. Thoughts are the products of our cognitive brain, the higher center that differentiates humans from all other forms of life. Mastery of our thoughts is undeniably linked with success. In order to deliver success, we must overcome a range of obstacles. The most powerful challenges come from within.

Our primitive brain stem is charged with the critical role of protecting us. It steers us powerfully to flight or fight. Its currency is fear. When we dream of success, the cautious voice of our primitive brain quickly answers with a dozen questions designed to protect us. "What if you fail? What if you lose all your money? What if you upset your friends? What if the world laughs at you? What if it's not meant to be? What if you're not strong enough, smart enough…?" The list is endless, and as we listen to our voice of caution, questions become doubts, and doubts become fears. *Belief* fades. Failure ensues.

Over time, if we heed the well-intentioned concerns of our primitive brain too often, our cognitive brain becomes contaminated with *limiting beliefs*. If we frequently give in to the doubt-filled question, "are you really brave enough?" we entrench in ourselves the limiting belief that we are, in fact, not brave enough. This may be a subtle shift, but it has a profound impact. When we incapacitate our cognitive brain with limiting beliefs, failure is inevitable. Instead of coming up with reasons to try, we come up with excuses not to.

Many of us enter adulthood with limiting beliefs swarming our minds. Kind parents have protected us from failure and pain. In their efforts to shield us, they seed limiting beliefs. They start by saying, "I don't want you to get hurt by taking on challenges that are too big for you," and end up entrenching in us the belief that life is filled with challenges bigger than we are. This is clearly a limiting belief. Or, in the interests of financial prudence, they ask if we think that "money grows on trees." Over time, we come to hold the belief that money is an elusive luxury that only the rich and famous deserve. Another limiting belief.

So how do we overcome these deeply entrenched and disempowering limiting beliefs?

First, we have to recognize the undermining fear. Each time we experience doubt, we must ask what is driving it. Is it driven by legitimate, rational, evidence-based argument? Or is it merely an excuse, fueled by a limiting belief? We must interrogate the fear, challenging it to defend itself and prove its factual base. In the absence of a watertight defense, the limiting belief is exposed for the excuse it really is, and progress is possible.

Then, free of the excuse, we can again invoke the power of the cognitive brain to redirect our creative energy toward the desired outcome: *belief.* The prevailing voices in our head become positive, and we are able to silence the protective cries of our primitive brain. Success follows.

How does this relate back to BodyWHealth?

First, the means for WHealth Seekers to succeed are entrenched in our biology. Understanding how the cognitive, emotional, and primitive brains interact helps us to coach them toward success. This is true throughout all aspects of life, including WHealth.

Second, it's important that we understand the limiting beliefs we hold about WHealth. Society teaches us that health fades as life progresses, that decay is inevitable. Why should we accept this? We have within our grasp the ability to resist decay and optimize our health. Society teaches us that only a few lucky people are happy through their lives, that the rest of us must struggle through constant uphill journeys. Why? What if we are destined to be one of the so-called "lucky few"? How would you live differently if you *knew* that you were one of those lucky ones? Well, here is the good news: *Belief* makes that possible.

Understand the limiting beliefs holding you back from the abundant WHealth you deserve. Employ your cognitive brain to promote powerful positive thought. Prepare for WHealth!

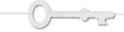

"You can, you should, and if you're brave enough to start, you will."

STEPHEN KING

YOUR PRESCRIPTION FOR WHEALTH

I have described the anatomy of *belief*, outlining the complex relationships that exist between the three layers of the human brain; the power of *belief*, the essential ingredient of any successful venture; and the limiting beliefs that can be roadblocks on your way to success. Now I want to show you how to train your brain to consistently plan, prepare for, and deliver success. When you *believe*, you will enjoy abundant WHealth!

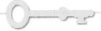

"Believe you can and you're halfway there."

THEODORE ROOSEVELT

Let's go back to where we started. We as human beings stood out from our mammalian peers when we added a massive cerebral cortex to our brains. This gigantic leap added thought and reason to our weaponry. The most obvious advantage this gives us is our problem-solving ability. We are able to apply complex intellectual reasoning to address challenges and create opportunities for success. For us to extract the full benefit of the huge selective advantage conferred on us by the cognitive layer of our brains, we need to engage it in liberating us from the restrictive *doubts* imposed by our primitive brains. We need to employ our cognitive powers to flood our brains with positive *ideas*, indirectly influencing and co-opting the emotional brain in such a way that our *desires* become so strong that they transform into *belief*. That's when we tap into the full power of the human brain. That's when we enjoy success. That is what every highly successful person has learned to do. And that is what WHealth Seekers must do, too.

Belief drives success, almost automatically. But in order for this to happen, *belief* needs to be transformed into appropriate actions, and those actions need to overcome both expected and unexpected obstacles. This doesn't happen in a flash; it takes time. But *belief* is the fuel for this process. It provides the energy, the resilience, the patience, and the strength required to get the job done. The fact that it takes time makes it harder. A moment of *belief* is easy. I have them all the time—often at two o'clock in the morning! But by the time I wake up to shower and dress, my trusty reptilian brain has generously offered to protect me from the pain of failure and once again flooded my cognitive and emotional brains with doubt. Like me, you may have to work to actively uphold your *belief* for a long time in order to deliver success. Successful men and women know how to do this.

Study any highly successful person, and you'll find that *belief* is the secret behind his or her accomplishment. Nelson Mandela lived behind bars for twenty-seven years, never giving up hope for a free and fair South Africa, because he *believed*. Neil Armstrong took his "small step for man" and "giant step for mankind" because he and his NASA colleagues *believed*. Helen Keller would not let the loss of two senses (sight and sound) stop her from becoming a highly impactful sociopolitical activist, because she *believed*. Charismatic British billionaire Sir Richard Branson turned a tiny student newspaper into a leading record label and then a megacorporation that includes his flagship Virgin Atlantic Airways, because he *believed unrelentingly* in his vision.

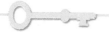

"You are essentially who you create yourself to be, and all that occurs in your life is the result of your own making."

STEPHEN RICHARDS

SIMPLE RECOMMENDATIONS FOR **BELIEVING**

1. *Think positively.* It sounds so easy, right? Scientists call this *autosuggestion*. We know that we control the cognitive brain. We know that the cognitive brain influences the emotional brain and is able to override the primitive brain. Use this knowledge. Flood your brain with positive statements about your inevitable success. Repeat them over and over again. We know that the cognitive brain can fall victim to the primitive brain's repetitive messages of doubt and fear; it is highly susceptible to them. Use autosuggestion to ensure that your cognitive brain is teeming with positive thoughts. If your reptilian brain can seize the autopilot and drive you toward failure, then you can just as easily grab the controls and drive toward success instead.

2. *Understand and accept the voice of your primitive brain, without legitimizing it.* This is a critically important nuance of your overall success. You have now learned about the existence of your primitive brain, and understand that it is an important part of who you are. It protects you from catastrophe. Respect it. Understand its role. Accept that it will (and should) always have an opinion. But *do not* give it too much attention. It is much like a whiny child; you have to take heed of it. But take only a quick look to see that there is no major disaster that you have overlooked, and then ignore it. Attention reinforces bad behavior. Distract and, if necessary, overwhelm it with positive thoughts!

3. *Empathize with your idea.* Olympic champions do this when they practice visualization. They spend long hours building the complete image of success in their minds, using all their senses. Spend time building the mental image of success until you can see, hear, taste, smell, and feel it vividly in your mind.

4. *Repeat your rhetoric.* Your positive rhetoric must be a daily habit, put into action throughout the day. Write your success statement down. Learn it by heart. Say it out loud. Turn it into a song and sing it. Paste it on your wall, your ceiling, or your steering wheel. Keep it alive.

5. *Surround yourself with positive people.* If you don't have them, search for them, find them, and embrace them. Every positive echo of your positive thoughts is like gold. "Can-do" is infectious—contagious, actually.

6. *Avoid negative people.* In fact, run from them. The voice of your primitive brain is loud enough. You don't need a team of naysayers augmenting these undermining pulls.

7. *Practice.* For many of us, the habit of positive thinking and *belief* is new or underdeveloped. Practice on small things every day.

8. *Move along the action verb list.* Success is no accident; it's a deliberate journey. Track your progress actively. You may move backward and forward along this continuum. That's okay. Write down where you are today, and use the power of your cognitive brain to ensure that your entire being moves toward anticipating success.

> Imagine... Want... Desire... Believe... Plan... Act...
> Expect... Demand... Anticipate... Celebrate!

9. *Do first the things you're avoiding most.* I love this little tip. If you're unsure where the voice of doubt is hurting you most, pull out your to-do list. Look at those items that slide from day to day. I bet you'll find they're often the most important tasks! The things you dread bring you closest to your inner doubt, face to face with your reptilian brain. It's understandable that you want to stay away from this monster, but don't give it the upper hand. We often overestimate the time required for unpalatable tasks, justifying our procrastination by saying that we'll get to them when we have the time. Turn them into ten-minute challenges. You'll be surprised how many of them start to disappear with a few minutes of concerted effort.

10. *Fake it to make it.* In the early stages of building *belief,* you might have a desire that is not quite ready to be a belief. That's okay, but keep the struggle internal. On the outside, project the success that you desire. The act of designing, building, and maintaining your "game face" is a powerful, reinforcing cognitive discipline, and there is some very elegant science that proves its value.

CONCLUSION

Three decades ago I was a very young doctor. I was on my first rotation in a surgical unit. As was customary, when I joined the team, I took over a list of patients who would be my primary responsibility. On that list was a man I shall never forget. Together, we learned one of life's greatest lessons.

John was about twenty-five years old. He was intelligent and likeable. He came from a very underprivileged background. He had grown up on the dirty, dangerous streets of an African township. He had applied himself to his studies in a grossly under-resourced school, and had secured a reliable income working for a small company in the city.

I walked up to his bed on that first day. His eyes and face shifted toward me, eager to find his new caregiver. They offered me a warm welcome, even as they hinted at the apprehension implicit in a new beginning.

His eyes and smile were the only flicker of life in his body.

John's medical journey had started on a dark and dangerous evening. He got off his train at the same time he always had, moving fast through the shadows, eager to get home to his modest dwelling where he knew his sister would be waiting with a warm meal. He would eat quickly, then collapse into bed to sleep before rising again at four o'clock the next morning, in time to get back to work in the city.

But this night was different. They were waiting for him at his home, with guns. They had elected not to labor as most people do, but had chosen instead to prey on honest, hardworking folk to feed their own needs. These thugs knew he had some money—not much, but they wanted it.

John turned to face them, willing to give up his own life to protect his sister if need be. The staccato fire of an AK-47 shattered the night as several rounds entered his chest and abdomen. Miraculously, they did minor harm—nothing that two operations couldn't fix. But the single bullet that penetrated his spinal column, smashing the vertebrae and severing his spinal cord, left him a quadriplegic for life.

I shook John's lifeless hand. The odor of decay hung heavily on the air. I knew that he had been lying like this, flat on his back, for months. Overworked nursing staff did their best to protect him from bedsores and the decay of physical inactivity. But biology was stronger than their meager resources. I knew that we would have to take him back into the operating room soon to clean up those deep, festering wounds, before returning him to the inevitable doom of his hospital bed.

It took me a few days to get to know John. He had been put into a remote corner of the surgical unit, allowing the dedicated nursing staff to attend to more urgent patients. I would visit him twice a day as I did my rounds, choosing to sit on his bed, looking into his hungry eyes. Somehow, he'd kept a tiny sparkle in them despite the miserable fate that he'd been allotted. I would talk with him. My voice and his eyes. Somehow, we connected.

After a week, my responsibility became clear to me. At the end of an all-night shift where we saved and lost the lives of others caught in the same web of violence, I stopped at his bed. The charge nurse and her entourage stood with me as I looked John in the eye and said, "You're going home. Not today, or even tomorrow, but soon."

It was clear to me that the hospital was the worst place for him. He was better off in the care of his sister in a dark room on the dangerous streets than he was trapped in his body in a sterile hospital room.

John's eyes froze with fear. The nursing staff—all experienced, caring people—fell silent. Time stood still for a few brief seconds in that crazy, turbulent space. A tear welled up in the corner of his eye and tricked slowly down onto his pillow.

The next few weeks were filled with frenetic activity. Initially, the entire nursing staff stood against me. I arrived at work the next day to have the hospital superintendent meet me, to dissuade me from my plan. But I was unwavering. I *believed* that John could do it. We brought in his sister. She was strong, smart, neat, and fastidious. She learned about wound care and mobilization. Slowly, John's gaze went from fearful to hopeful. Before long, I saw a rampant fire of determination and *belief* in him.

Finally, the day arrived. I had tears in my eyes as I said goodbye to John and loaded him into the back of the ambulance that would carry him home. As they drove him away into the chaos of the sprawling shantytown, I stood for a long time, holding my breath.

Four weeks later, I was examining another post-surgical patient in our outpatient department. I was updating her follow-up instructions when a loud noise disrupted the entire building. People were shouting, clapping, and singing. I pulled back the curtain of the examination cubicle to see a throng of nurses and patients dancing their way into the clinic. At their center, John sat upright in his wheelchair. He grinned broadly, and tears streamed down his cheeks. I could see that he was well, life radiating from his face.

We had done it! My *belief* became his *belief*. My nursing colleagues and social workers joined us with their *belief*. Together, we had mounted a formidable campaign against seemingly insurmountable odds, conquered fear, and delivered a life-changing outcome.

Thank you, John, for sharing with me this profound lesson in *belief*.

I hope that you now understand the magic of your brain. We respect that the primitive brain is there to keep us safe. We need and appreciate this, but at the same time know that this can be a source of fear and doubt that handicaps us from reaching our goals. We understand that the combined power of the cognitive and emotional brains in generating *belief* is so strong that it overcomes these fears. When *belief* prevails, action and success follow.

The theory is simple, but putting this knowledge to work in your life is far from easy. You need to practice *belief* every day. This is the hard work that paves the road to success.

When you achieve *belief*, profound faith in your dream, you will be flooded with transformative power. WHealth will follow.

I leave you with the Ralph Waldo Emerson quote again, this time with nuanced emphasis. Your future is in your hands. You *are* going to become someone; that is guaranteed. The beauty is that *you* get to choose who that person is!

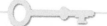

"The ONLY person you are destined to become
is the person YOU decide to be."

RALPH WALDO EMERSON

WHealth Plus

In addition to flooding your brain with positive ideas to cultivate *belief* in and for yourself, I advocate that you optimize your posture to drive *belief*, employ the power of *belief* during tough times, and introduce *belief* to your family. You will be amazed at the meaningful impact these *belief* expansions will have on your WHealth journey.

THE POWER OF STANDING TALL: A SIMPLE RECIPE FOR BELIEF

Belief is the precursor to success. Great people across the ages have all known this powerful secret. Each one of us has the right to achieve success in our lives, and the ability to learn to *believe*. This is the path to BodyWHealth. Here is one simple way to engage your body to launch you toward success.

Early in our development, we learn to read body language. Even before we can understand spoken language, we react to the touch and gestures of our parents and families. Only later do we learn what their words mean. Deep inside, our brains are constantly observing and reacting to nonverbal cues from the people we interact with. But what about our own body language? How does our brain react to that?

Picture two separate moments in your life. Start with a low point. Visualize yourself at a time when your mind was filled with doubt and fear. See yourself in detail in the theater of your mind. What do you see? You were small, hunched, and closed. Your voice and nonverbal gestures were modest. You shuffled along with cautious little steps.

Now transport yourself rapidly to a moment of success, a triumphal event where your mind was filled with elation and pride. Again, picture yourself. How did you appear to the world? You stood tall and open. Your head was high and your shoulders back. You may even have raised both arms above your head in the broad V for victory. Your stride was long and meaningful.

Your voice was strong and your gestures generous.

We know that our bodies mirror our feelings. When you were afraid, your body shrunk away from the world. When you were successful, your body expanded and you stood tall with pride. Our body language is highly responsive to our emotional state. But what about the inverse? Might our brain actually listen to our body language, too?

Science is beginning to answer this question for us, and the conclusions are robust and exciting. Here is the compelling truth: Our brains watch our body language and learn from it. When we act powerless, we become powerless. But the even more valuable truth in this same observation is that when we act powerful, we become powerful!

Researchers have shown how we are able to change our mindset by changing our posture—and it all started with a smile. Many years ago, social scientists asked people to put a pencil into their mouths. Simply by holding the pencil horizontally between their lips in a manner that forced a smile, the study participants became happy! Nothing changed for these people except that their face was forced into a smile…and they became happier.

Two critical hormones mediate the balance of confidence we enjoy in our lives. Testosterone is the hormone of positivity and power (both men and women have it, but at different concentrations). Cortisol is the stress hormone of negativity and doubt. Powerful, successful people tend to have higher levels of testosterone and lower levels of cortisol.

And here is the liberating science regarding those hormones: If you adopt a power pose (standing tall, with head up, shoulders back, and arms high in a V for victory) for as little as two minutes, you increase the levels of testosterone in your blood and decrease the levels of cortisol. Your brain senses these changes, and your level of self-belief rises! Researchers have demonstrated in several different situations and studies how this simple act not only improves your own belief, but also how it spills out to influence those around you. When *you believe* and *they believe*, success flows!

Amy Cuddy, a social scientist from Harvard, recommends a simple, two-minute daily ritual to tap into this power. Stand tall with an open body in an explicit power pose for two minutes every day. Allow your brain to enjoy the boost of testosterone and reduced levels of cortisol, and you will *believe*.

Do this before important meetings, sporting events, or performances, and your elevated self-confidence will translate into enhanced performance—and greater WHealth.

For many years, personal coaches have advocated that their clients "fake it until they make it." We have now substantiated the science behind this concept. Amy Cuddy phrases it slightly differently: "Fake it until you *believe* it. Our bodies change our minds." When you *believe* it, you will make it.

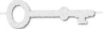

> *"Whatever the mind can conceive and believe,*
> *the mind can achieve."*
>
> NAPOLEON HILL

THE POWER OF PERSISTENCE: SURVIVING TOUGH TIMES

BodyWHealth is the reward for a life of healthy habit, fueled by persistence and resilience. The easy days are easy; true wisdom and courage come from thriving on the tough days. But how do you get through those difficult times? I'd like to take a little excursion with you to permit you to see the power of *belief* at work.

I love the ocean. She heals and refreshes me. She gives me energy and ideas. I am in awe of her power, her breadth and depth, and her many faces. I admire and respect the brave men and women who study her and work to protect her. I am part of the extensive kindred spirits who love to play in her, and will take any excuse to swim, dive, surf, or kayak. More than anything else, I am respectful of her immense strength, most evident in the towering waves that crash relentlessly on the beaches and rocks of our continents.

My fascination with waves sometimes leads me to explore dangerous places. Huge waves tend to attract a tiny group of adventurers, lured by the might of the ocean and the thrill of participating in her spectacular displays. Now, don't get me wrong, I haven't surfed or swum in 100-foot waves (yet). Maybe one day, but for now, I am drawn simply by the spectacle, and the brave athletes who test their skills and courage in these supernatural forces.

I recently met a veteran big wave surfer. Many people thrill in watching online videos and photographs of these brave athletes surfing down a wall of water, escaping the thunderous crest that threatens to deluge them with tons of churning water. It is easy to understand the elation that drives them to stare danger in the face. My interest, though, is in how they survive the long, terrifying moments when things go wrong—when the world turns into a boiling mass of water, pounding them and sucking them in different directions while trying to crush them under its weight, and sometimes against a rocky shore.

I was fascinated by the surfer's responses to my questions. He told me that big wave surfers train themselves to hold a calming image in their minds. When things get really rough, and it seems like they may have to hold their breath for eternity, and they feel like they're down to their last drop of oxygen, they bring those images into their minds. It's an emotional parachute.

This made so much sense to me in the context of the underlying neuroscience of our brains. As you know, danger activates our primitive brains to flood our bodies with adrenaline and other chemicals that evoke powerful fight or flight responses. If left alone, our body responds dutifully in frantic activity to preserve life. This is a major problem if you're going to be underwater for a prolonged period of time. Your heart races, your limbs thrash, and your body craves the very precious oxygen that you're burning excessively in your frenzy. Your lungs are desperate for air, but if you inhale, you will drown. Signals from the primitive brain also jolt the emotional brain into action. Fear becomes panic, compounding your risk and exacerbating the red haze that threatens your mind.

But remember that Mother Nature has gifted humans with a massive cerebral cortex—the thinking part of our brains. Powerfully, she has established dominance of this cognitive brain over our primitive and emotional brains. The cognitive brain is under our voluntary control. At will, we are able to override the urgent clamors of the primitive and emotional brains using powerful positive thoughts.

That is exactly what these big wave surfers train themselves to do. When panic threatens to condemn them to a watery death, they invoke the override of their cognitive brains. Holding on to the tranquil image of a peaceful landscape, or the reassuring face of a loved one or their favorite pet, they breathe calm into their minds. In this more relaxed state, they are able to hold their breath, stop thrashing, regain their gravitational bearings, and eventually surface to gulp in delicious oxygen-rich air again.

Perhaps you've never dived under a big wave in the ocean, and never tasted that particular fear. But I'm sure that you will recognize the idea of overwhelming feelings of panic and confusion. You have undoubtedly experienced these in many different ways throughout your life. Use your understanding of the neuroscience of the brain, and train yourself like a big wave surfer. Each of us should have a beautiful, peaceful image in the back of our minds that we can reach for in moments of rage or panic. Find one, and practice bringing it into the front of your mind on good days. Then put it into practice on the bad days. Recall your image when your boss criticizes you, your spouse yells at you, or your children fight with each other. Do it when you have to pay the hefty tax bill you hadn't anticipated or when you receive bad news. Increasingly, you will be able to use this new skill on the tough days, getting you through the terrifying turbulence until you can surface to gulp in fresh air again. This will empower you on your BodyWHealth journey.

THE POWER OF ROYALTY: MY PLEA TO ALL PARENTS

Investing in the WHealth of your children is one of the most important transactions you'll ever make. Parents of young children often ask me what they should do to raise confident, successful, WHealthy young men and women. Here is what I tell them, based on my understanding of the neuroscience of the human brain and the power of *belief*: "Treat them like royals!"

To help these parents understand further, I ask them to enter the theater of their imagination and picture their children dressed as young members of a royal family on an important day. Picture them standing on a castle balcony overlooking a crowded square filled with adoring subjects. Picture them walking with their family amongst the crowd, heads high, with a self-assured gait. Their faces, body language, and behavior ooze confidence. The world is theirs, and they can choose their own futures.

The human brain works in a wonderful way. If our brain is filled with positive thoughts that resonate with our emotional desires, *belief* flows easily and naturally. The royal child hears affirmation at every corner. The whole world shouts out, "you are worthy!" Their ears faithfully pass the message on to their brains, in particular to their cognitive brains. Their cognitive brains hear this message hour after hour, day after day. It becomes deeply ingrained in their being, and they *believe*.

Because they *believe*, they walk tall and think big. They don't hear the nagging voice of their primitive brains urging caution as we do. Its paltry efforts are dwarfed by the resounding echoes in their cognitive brain—"You are worthy; you are worthy" becomes "I am worthy; I am worthy..."—and thought becomes *belief*, which becomes actions and success. It's a simple recipe.

Most of us don't have royal fans and an entourage supplying the constant affirmation that royals enjoy. That's where we step in as parents. Our voices have to become the affirmation of the masses for our children. Our voices have to shout loudly, every hour of every day, "you are worthy; you are worthy; you are worthy!"

My only word of caution is that even as you soak their growing brains in the "you are worthy" message, it must be balanced with the twin guidance that it is hard work that will be the forerunner of their success. Self-worthiness in the absence of hard work is *entitlement*, a dangerous affliction for royals and lesser mortals alike.

Finally, the grand challenge for every parent is that we have to model royal behavior for our children. We have to model self-belief and self-worth. And in doing so, we will help not only our children but also ourselves to develop an incredible capacity for *belief*. A family who *believes* together is a WHealthy family indeed.

THE ROAD TO ENABLING MINDSETS

Enabling mindsets empower you to pursue WHealthy behaviors toward your final goal of BodyWHealth. Making no excuses, developing WHealthy habits, and *believing* in yourself are vital to your success as a WHealth Seeker.

Affirmation and gratitude are powerful forces on your journey. As we pause on our journey together, please celebrate with me the fantastic progress you've made toward WHealth. I hope you will allow me to share my own appreciation.

My Gratitude List

Thank you for reading this book.

Thank you for learning that exercise is the cornerstone of BodyWHealth, and that 10,000 steps on at least five days of each week will launch you on a transformative journey.

Thank you for appreciating the importance of energy balance and for counting calories to control your body fat reserves and limit the factory of inflammation that robs you of your WHealth.

Thank you for understanding that sleep restores physical (and emotional) WHealth, and that stress undermines both.

Thank you for eliminating excuses, for understanding the neuroscience of habit, and for establishing WHealthy patterns.

Thank you for *believing*!

CONCLUSION

It is now time to reach higher, to advance up the ladder toward the fullest expression of WHealth. Depending on where you started your journey, and how fast you are reading this book, you may not yet have the rewards of the physical foundation. That's okay. Even as you continue to build your physical base with diligence, patience, and joy, I invite you to move forward with me to explore and unlock the abundant riches of emotional WHealth.

WHealth
UNLOCKED
BEYOND PHYSICAL WHEALTH

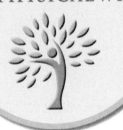

The beauty of your early journey—the first three Keys, which unlock physical WHealth—is its simplicity. Your path is linear, building on exercise to balance calories, then to sleep well, then to limit stress. This is how my own personal journey to WHealth started. As a physician and scientist, I found the early, physical journey predictable. And then to my utter amazement, as I started to restore my physical condition, I began to unlock unseen links between body, mind, and emotion. As I conquered excuses, developed WHealthy habits, and *believed*, happiness somehow found its way into my life, uninvited. This is the indescribable magic of BodyWHealth.

Your path is about to explode into a myriad of exciting opportunities. The journey beyond physical WHealth is a treasure trove of riches. My hope for you is that you will run through the orchard of emotional WHealth like an excited child, without fear of judgment, from tree to tree with sweet juices dripping off your chin.

Embrace your childlike courage and innocence; ignore the voice of caution—that inner serpent that fears embarrassment or, worse, doubts your worthiness. This is now the journey to happiness. Your work on the physical foundation and enabling mindsets has already primed your biology. *Believe.* Joy and abundance are within your grasp. It's in *your* hands!

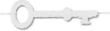

My hope for you is the inspiration and courage to look within, where each one of us holds the power to achieve abundant WHealth.

A Taste of Abundance

Your early work on the first three Keys to WHealth is an investment from which you're about to uncover tangible rewards. You will know from your own life that you can attain some of the riches of emotional WHealth even if your physical foundation is fragile. When my physical WHealth was at its lowest, I still enjoyed moments of happiness. In contrast, when your physical foundation is robust, emotional WHealth becomes more enduring, more pervasive, and without doubt, more alluring.

One of the many beauties of BodyWHealth is that the return on your investment grows disproportionally over time; its value compounds with your enduring effort. More than this, BodyWHealth becomes self-perpetuating after you pass a critical, invisible threshold—one you will recognize once you've crossed it. You will never forget the feeling of true WHealth once you have tasted it, and you are likely to continue to strive for more.

In her wisdom, Mother Nature designed irresistible chemical seduction for WHealthy behavior. The liberating joy of WHealth is underpinned by hormonal and chemical changes in our brains that we will explore in some detail in this section. From an evolutionary perspective, these adaptive behaviors increase our chance of success as individuals and as a species. Like physical WHealth, it is very clear that emotional WHealth is both a reward and an incentive.

When you have tasted WHealth, you not only crave more, but you are better equipped to deliver more to yourself. You know how to build WHealth, and you know that it is a highly valuable asset that will erode with neglect. You are a smarter, more devoted, and more motivated investor. You have both knowledge and experience. Subsequent investments have better returns. This is one of the principal reasons I advocate for a minimum investment of nine months (seven days, plus seven weeks, plus seven months). It not only entrenches life-changing habits, but it gives the owner of the Body a taste of abundant WHealth!

And that is the beauty of BodyWHealth, particularly when compared with wealth. There are fundamental differences between wealth and WHealth that makes the latter a more attractive investment. Concentration of wealth (the rich getting richer) thrives in the presence of underlying economic inequality. Economists would likely argue that global wealth is finite, leaving each of us competing for our share of the collective treasure. On the other hand, WHealth is an underexploited capability and reward that resides within each of us. We all have capacity for enormous expansion of individual WHealth. It is perhaps the perfect economy: Success breeds success, hard workers are rewarded disproportionately (the free-market principle), and there is equal access for all.

It's time for us to now extend our journey beyond physical WHealth. In this section of the book, we will focus on two central themes: *social engagement* and *purpose*. Mastery of these two intentions (spelled out in the final two Keys) will carry you deep into the land of plenty. Your reward will be enduring abundance and gratitude. This is BodyWHealth.

Whereas physical WHealth is a linear progression, starting with exercise and followed by balancing calories, sleeping well, and controlling stress, emotional WHealth is more expansive, even adventurous in nature. Physical WHealth is like the strong trunk of a tree that forms the supportive foundation for the emotionally WHealthy branches above, which in turn bear fruit and flowers, reaching wide to expose their precious treasures to life-giving sunlight.

You will notice a corresponding shift in the style of this book. The sections on physical WHealth and enabling mindsets end with prescriptions for specific actions. In this section, we explore emotional WHealth in a more liberal, adventurous framework. While I will still suggest activities and steps you might wish to take in your pursuit of happiness, I invite you to journey with me, exploring the many facets of emotional WHealth in a less structured manner. I hope that you will return often, as you discover and enjoy the abundant riches in your emotional orchard.

THE POWER OF THE EMOTIONAL BRAIN

We've talked a lot about the power of the cognitive brain, particularly in its ability to help us *believe*. But I'd like to focus now on the power of the emotional brain. Mother Nature, in her genius, embedded magic in the configuration of our central nervous system—magic that both incents and rewards the very behavior that makes us successful as individuals and as a species. That magic is called "happiness," and it has deep biological roots. Not surprisingly, it is intimately woven into the functioning of the emotional brain.

We are all in search of happiness, appropriately so. It is so universally important that the United Nations has declared an International Day of Happiness (March 20). The word "happiness" has many synonyms, partly reflecting the difficult nature of defining such an abstract phenomenon; partly reflecting the intensely personal, subjective quantification of the concept; and partly reflecting the range of intensity in this state.

Common to all definitions of happiness is that it is both mental and emotional in nature, and that it is characterized by positive, pleasurable emotions and thoughts. There is a range in the intensity of the state, with the mental and emotional components shifting independently of each other, resulting in a multitude of synonyms across two dimensions, as you can see below.

THE FULL RANGE OF HAPPINESS

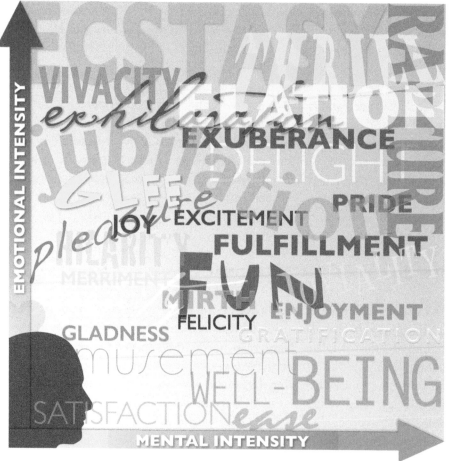

Like many other scientists, I have chosen the blanket term "happiness" to represent the full mental and emotional ranges of this state that is our common navigational beacon, the destination of our hunger and desire. This desire is deeply grounded in our biology, forged in the fires of our evolutionary past. It is an inescapable part of the human state—and thus, emotion is as central to our WHealth as is our physical well-being.

To understand this, we need to refresh our understanding of the developmental origins of our spectacular brains.

You will remember that we have a highly evolved, complex brain with three major components. At the center of our brain is the primitive (reptilian) brain. This was the earliest part of our brain to form, and it serves as our survival center, coordinating nervous activity that drives the fight and flight responses, protecting us from real and perceived danger. Next came the emotional brain. It is a collection of nerve centers, also known as the limbic system, and is responsible for our emotions. Finally, the third and outermost layer of our brain formed; it is the cerebral cortex, or cognitive brain. This massive addition is the seat of our advanced intellectual processing, and it enables us to include thought and reason in our mental arsenal.

When we explored the power of *belief*, we explored the interrelationships between these three layers of the brain. The cognitive brain is the only part under our direct, voluntary control, and it has the potential to influence both the emotional and the primitive brains. Similarly, although not within our direct control, the emotional brain can also influence the primitive brain. Hence, belief is the overall state of mind when a powerful thought from the cognitive brain, coupled with significant desire from the emotional brain, overcomes the doubt and fear generated in the primitive brain. I hope that you have practiced the power of *belief* in your life since you read about it in the previous section.

The addition of the emotional brain confers two distinct advantages to all animals that have it, differentiating us forever from creatures with less developed brains.

First, we have the ability to nurture our young. The cold reptilian brain does not equip its owner for this. Reptiles protect their young to only a limited extent, largely leaving them to survive on their own. The odds are stacked against any single individual surviving, so reptiles have multiple offspring in order to perpetuate the species. With the introduction of love and affection, by contrast, the emotional brain ensures that its owner invests deeply in the nurturing of its offspring. It takes a great deal of time and energy to grow and raise a complex mammal, so we with emotional brains have fewer young at any one time and apply all our energy and efforts to helping them on their path to adulthood.

Second, we forge constructive relationships with other members of our species in order to improve our individual and collective chances of success. The reptilian brain equips its landlords for limited interdependence with other adults of the same species, but the emotional brain endows consistent, valuable collaborative instincts to its mammalian owners. The emotional brain provides us with the power of affection, and we invest in fruitful and efficient relationships within our species and beyond. It's a huge quantum leap over less developed species.

So, how did Mother Nature decide to grant us these two massive gains? She carefully constructed the "hardware" (brain structure) and "software" (neurochemistry) of the emotional brain to both incent and reward nurturing and collaborative behavior.

Let's start with the hardware. Modern technology allows us to study brain activity during its routine functioning. If we watch which centers of the brain "light up" on an MRI, we can draw inferences about the physical location of specific brain functions. As a result of such brain studies, we know three important facts about the wiring of the emotional brain.

First, we know that both physical and emotional pain are processed in the same brain centers. In other words, our *physical* pain centers light up when we feel *emotional* pain. That explains how you can feel hollow, aching emotional pain as a real physical sensation when something terrible happens to you, such as in times of bereavement and loss. Emotional pain is *real* pain!

Perhaps more extraordinary is the fact that we appear to feel others' emotional pain in the same way we feel our own. The nerve centers that register pain when *we* are upset also light up when other people around us are distressed. What a powerful way to ensure empathy—we physically feel and experience the emotional pain of others as if it were our own pain!

NATURE'S GIFT: THE EMOTIONAL BRAIN

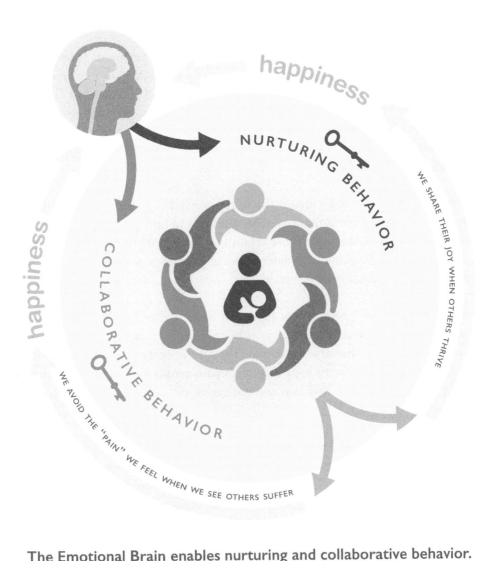

The Emotional Brain enables nurturing and collaborative behavior.
When we do these, we unlock happiness.

And finally, it appears that imaginary pain is centered in the same regions of the brain as real pain, explaining how the anticipation of loss can be as painful as loss itself.

The connection between the physical and the emotional realms of pain drives us to avoid emotional pain. We work to avoid emotional pain in ourselves, and we also work to avoid emotional pain in those who surround us. To do this, we care for them, we protect them, we guide them, we support them, and we comfort them. That's exactly what Mother Nature wanted us to do. That's why she gifted us with an emotional brain in the first place: to create loving community.

It is worth pausing to wonder at this exceptional design. Nature has gifted us with emotional brains that both link our body to our mind and emotions, and link us inescapably with those around us. We ignore these truths at our peril. Understanding this intention enables us to honor our design, unlocking the treasures of emotional WHealth.

Some scientists still believe that pain avoidance is the only motivation for our behavior. If the absence of pain is happiness, then avoiding pain is the path to happiness. For the most part, though, scientists are beginning to agree that there is more to happiness than pain avoidance. The clues to this lie in the chemistry of the brain and the causal relationship between "good acts" and happiness.

Beyond our basic brain hardware, Mother Nature also introduced several powerful chemical mediators into our brains to function as a sort of software. In particular, serotonin (5-hydroxytryptamine, or 5-HT) is believed to play a critical role in happiness. Serotonin is a neurotransmitter, connecting nerve cells with chemical bridges to allow transmission of signals from one nerve to the next. Serotonin is affectionately known as the "feel-good hormone" due to its role in regulating mood, appetite, and sleep (see how these all keep coming together?). We will explore other chemicals later (such as dopamine, *oxytocin*, and endorphins), but for now it's enough to know that there are several chemicals involved in happiness, and they work together to incent and reward "good" behavior.

What is "good" behavior? Mother Nature wanted to encourage nurturing and collaborative conduct among mammals, so she built a system wherein behavior and actions that foster nurturing and collaboration trigger the release of these chemical prizes. When your brain is flooded with serotonin, you feel the golden glow that you recognize as happiness. These chemicals become both the incentive and the reward. We are drawn to the biologically positive pro-social behaviors that light up the serotonin reward system. When we have that serotonin flowing, life feels good.

Unfortunately, we don't always heed the call of nature, and there are also diseases such as depression that seem to compromise the serotonin reward system. In both of those cases, we suffer the consequences. In the absence of happiness, the world becomes a dark and lonely place. There are both emotional and physical consequences for us, beyond just mood disruption. Sadness (a term I use loosely to describe the absence of happiness) is associated with physical disease such as heart disease, stroke, diabetes, and premature death.

A seminal study conducted by scientists from Yale and the University of California, Berkeley, showed how isolated older individuals were two to three times more vulnerable to premature death than their age-matched peers with extensive interpersonal connectivity.[47] Another study by Harvard and University of Pittsburgh scientists evaluated more than 6,000 subjects from several large national databases over a fifteen-year period, and found that emotional vitality appeared to reduce the risk of coronary disease.[48] Happiness has been shown to both prolong life and improve quality of life, partly through reducing the risk of the same diseases that sadness causes.

Now here is the real magic of the emotional brain: Just as we learned to activate the overriding influence of the cognitive brain to drive belief, so we can use our cognitive brains to positively influence our emotional brains in driving happiness. This is the path to emotional WHealth. While there appears to be some genetic and familial predisposition to this happiness-inducing competence, it remains a faculty that we can *all* activate and enhance!

Let me repeat that: While some people appear to have a naturally happy disposition, we *all* have the power to unlock our own happiness. The privilege of the human condition is that we can engage our powerful cognitive brains to guide and nurture our emotional brains. Your happiness is in *your own* hands!

THE PILLARS OF HAPPINESS: ENGAGEMENT AND PURPOSE

The science of happiness is emerging as a flourishing discipline. Leading universities now devote resources to mind-body medicine, and government and private sources are funding research to understand the origins and impact of happiness.

The Grant Study and the parallel Glueck Study, both conducted by Harvard scientists, have followed two cohorts of men across more than seventy-five years. The two studies together include men from a range of socioeconomic and educational backgrounds. The objective of the research was to define predictors of healthy aging: in other words, to discover the secrets to a happy and successful life. The research findings have been published in three books, the most recent titled *Triumphs of Experience*,[49] by lead author George Vaillant. Although the study included only men, a limitation resulting from the antiquated gender bias prevalent when the research started, it nevertheless has conclusions that have been verified in subsequent, more fully representative work. The power of the original Harvard research is its incredible duration, providing illuminating windows into the full lifetimes of the participants.

Two findings stand out above all others from this work, and have been reinforced through many other studies, leading us to the remaining two Keys to WHealth.

The first finding is that *social engagement* (Key #6) is a fundamental pillar of happiness. It trumped career success, financial success, and physical health as the top driver of happiness. The others play important roles, to be sure, but they are dwarfed by the critical role of interpersonal connectivity in driving emotional health and success. We flourish in the presence of supportive, loving relationships. Interestingly, intelligence was insignificant as a driver of happiness, and above a certain level of intellectual competence, it played no role at all. This leaves us squarely focused on the critical role of the emotional brain in driving full WHealth.

The second pillar of happiness emerging from this and other research is the role of *purpose* (Key #7). This links closely with Nature's requirement of us to nurture our children and to collaborate fruitfully with others. Clearly, when we are focused on our role as contributors in society, we are rewarded with the neurochemical prize of happiness (and physical health, too).

Emotional WHealth Flourishes
Off a Robust Foundation of Physical WHealth

The branches of Social Engagement and Purposeful Living support the abundant fruits of Emotional WHealth.

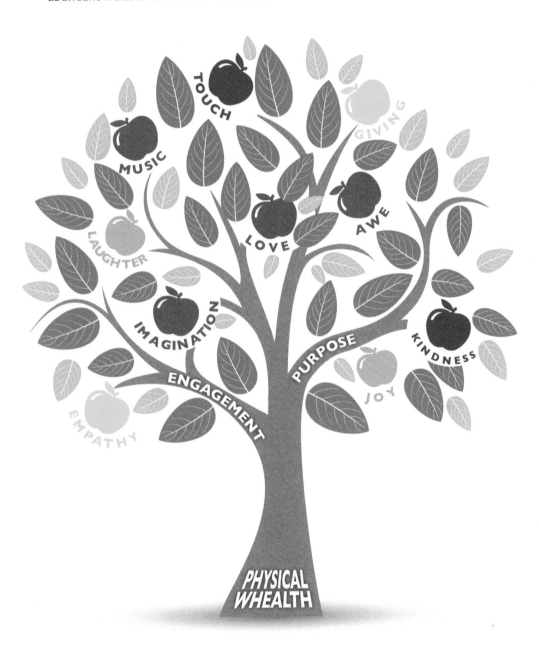

Two other important characteristics of happiness emerge from the social sciences to inspire us to work on our own happiness. The first is that happiness is an elastic phenomenon—we can always enhance it. In fact, some of the men who started with the worst-looking happiness profiles early in the Grant study ended up being the happiest. Employing the Keys of social engagement and purpose can powerfully influence our futures, at any age. Secondly, the challenges and obstacles we face on our journey need not divert us away from happiness. Rather, the way we handle adversity and challenge can propel us further up the ladder of happiness. Professor Vaillant cites the example of Mother Teresa, who survived an unfortunate early life. Instead of being consumed by her own emotional strife, an outward focus of creativity and care propelled her to an enormous humanitarian contribution. In the case of Mother Teresa, and each of us, the principles of social engagement and purpose emerge as critical drivers of happiness and success.

We're at the gates to the orchard of emotional WHealth. Nature has gifted you with the keys to unlock the gate and to explore the abundance beyond. Please join me—it's time to move forward again. I share the same joy and wonder in accompanying you on your adventure as I felt opening the gates to my own orchard several years ago.

KEY #6: INVEST SOCIALLY

Engage abundantly in your relationships.

Social engagement has powerful impact on both longevity and health.

You may recall me mentioning the 1978 study conducted by scientists from Yale and the University of California, Berkeley, showing how isolated older individuals were two to three times more vulnerable to premature death than their socially active peers.[50] Another group of scientists from Brigham Young University and the University of North Carolina pooled the data from 148 studies, together including over 300,000 participants and conducted over three decades.[51] The results were entirely aligned with the 1978 study, showing a 50 percent increased likelihood of survival for those with higher levels of social engagement, translating to an additional four years of life on average. This means that the added mortality risk of isolation is even higher than the risk associated with either physical inactivity or obesity.

The relationship between social connectivity and longevity is hard to define, but research into social engagement and health may give us some clues. Sheldon Cohen of the Carnegie Mellon University has pioneered research into the common cold.[52] In his collection of work, known as the "Pittsburgh Common Cold Studies," he and his colleagues have shown that stress (especially long-term stress) creates an increased susceptibility to the common cold. Not surprisingly, stress disrupts the immune system via pro-inflammatory cytokines. Remember the critical balance between the pro-inflammatory cytokines and the anti-inflammatory cytokines? Here they are at work again, with the bad guys dominating in stressful situations, resulting in negative physical consequences. But more importantly, Cohen and his colleagues have shown that social engagement reduces the risk of common cold infection, even in high-stress individuals. Warm, supportive relationships protect you by strengthening your immune system.

Janice Kiecolt-Glaser, professor of psychiatry at Ohio State University, and her colleague Ronald Glaser have devoted their careers to understanding the role of loneliness-induced stress in immune suppression.[53] In a range of research subjects including medical students taking exams, spouses before and after separation and divorce, and breast cancer survivors, they have shown how social isolation leaves us vulnerable to both infectious and metabolic disease.

Research has also demonstrated that blood pressure fluctuates in association with relationships. Close, supportive spousal and family relationships result in lower, healthier blood pressures. Another study by Harvard and University of Pittsburgh scientists evaluated more than 6,000 subjects from several large national databases over a fifteen-year period and found that emotional vitality appeared to reduce the risk of coronary disease.[54]

All of this research shows us that emotional and social engagement drives both health (by impacting the inflammatory cytokine balance favorably) and happiness (through serotonin levels in the brain). That is why the sixth Key to WHealth is all about investing socially: *Engage abundantly in your relationships*. In order to find happiness, we WHealth Seekers must engage socially as often as possible.

To Live, We Need (To) Love!

Loneliness is not only a sad place; it's a bad place. Research has shown that lonely people die prematurely. The magnitude of the risk is considerable. It's as bad as smoking! Loneliness impairs the immune system, triggers inflammation, and disrupts sleep. You know that inflammation increases the risk of heart disease, diabetes, and cancer, and you know that the quality of your sleep directly affects your BodyWHealth. So, loneliness is not only a sad place to be, it's also a profoundly unhealthy place to be.

More importantly, we know that it's not enough to simply *be* with people; you can be lonely in a big city, or in a marriage. You have to be *engaged* with them to enjoy WHealth. By now, you understand that this is programmed into our brains in both the hardware and the software.

Picture yourself in your most lonely, reactive, selfish, defensive state. Perhaps this sounds familiar. When you're in this state, you have retreated to your reptilian brain. Your survival instincts take over. It's cold, and it's isolated. It can also be a destructive, vicious downward spiral. Loneliness encourages you to retreat further into your reptilian brain, which makes you defensive and scared. In fear, you shun further contact and exaggerate your loneliness. This is a problem because we were not designed for either physical or emotional isolation.

Happily, Mother Nature gifted us with our emotional brains and the feel-good chemical serotonin as a pleasurable reward in order to reinforce social engagement. The emotional brain, with its serotonin treasure, is sandwiched between the primitive brain and the cognitive brain. It is subject to the influence of both. The primitive brain exerts a negative, selfish pressure, insisting that we survive. The cognitive brain is under our active control and can influence our emotions either positively or negatively. If we only had the primitive brain, we would be governed by fear and would live defensively. We often default to this mode under stress. The primitive brain is strong, but the emotional brain (and cognitive brain) can override its influence. Serotonin switches off adrenaline and cortisol secretion, opposing our primitive fight and flight response and enabling us to control our selfish instincts. Note that we oppose *fear* with *love*. This is the fundamental antithesis that governs our lives.

Several things are known to stimulate an increase in serotonin in your emotional brain. Physical contact is the most important. When you snuggle close to loved ones on a cold night (a good survival strategy for warm-blooded mammals), you are rewarded with a serotonin boost. Both affirmation and parenting behavior have also been shown to increase this feel-good neurotransmitter. Finally, we know that exercise and light increase serotonin levels. Just as our emotional brains crave all of these activities, so we need all of them for Body W Health.

In essence, we need fear to survive; but to *live*, we need *love*!

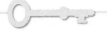

> *"Being deeply loved by someone gives you strength,*
> *while loving someone deeply gives you courage."*
>
> LAO TZU

GIVE TO RECEIVE: THE SCIENCE OF KINDNESS

Gifts never move in only one direction. That's the official word from social anthropologists. As in the laws of physics, every action has an equal and opposite reaction. The giver is always rewarded with return gifts of appreciation or respect. But that's not all. Giving drives tangible health benefits for the giver that are profound stepping-stones toward BodyWHealth.

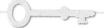

"We make a living by what we get,
but we make a life by what we give."

WINSTON CHURCHILL

Social contact is important, but we maximize our gains when we go beyond simple contact to engage empathetically with others. I propose that giving may be the most powerful form of social engagement, and there is good science to back this assertion.

The scientific name for giving is "pro-social behavior" and includes closely related concepts such as generosity and empathy. Scientists have demonstrated that we start our lives with an innate bias toward generosity.[55] Toddlers under the age of two are happier giving away treats than receiving them. More importantly, "costly" pro-social acts (generosity which disadvantages the giver), such as a toddler giving away his or her last treat, makes children happier than easy giving.

Giving is associated with happiness in adults, too. In their book *The Paradox of Generosity,*[56] sociologists Christian Smith and Hilary Davidson report that adults who describe themselves as very happy volunteer on average six hours of their time to good causes each month, while those who describe themselves as unhappy donate 90 percent less time. They also found depression prevalence 25 percent lower in adults who give away more than 10 percent of their disposable incomes.

Giving not only drives happiness, but it drives health, too. A provocative study published in 2013 in *JAMA Pediatrics* evaluated the health benefits of weekly community service in high school students.[57] After only four months, adolescents who gave their time to others lost weight while non-volunteers gained weight. More interesting to me is that the levels of the pro-inflammatory cytokine IL6 was lower in those who volunteered their time than in their peers. IL6 and excessive inflammation are implicated as mediators of serious diseases such as heart disease, diabetes, and even cancer. So, giving may offer dramatic long-term health benefits.

The value of giving is not limited to happiness and health. Early pro-social behavior in children has been shown to exert a strongly positive influence on subsequent academic performance and social development.[58]

How does this all work? Serotonin levels increase in the brain during social engagement and drive feelings of well-being. A different chemical, a hormone called oxytocin, has also been implicated in pro-social behavior.[59] Oxytocin is released when people are empathetic and generous. Moreover, the same hormone actually drives empathetic behavior. Oxytocin just happens to be the critical hormone involved in breast-feeding, a highly empathetic act of personal generosity. No small coincidence, I'm sure!

To make this science even more interesting, researchers at Harvard have shown that generosity becomes self-reinforcing.[60] Giving makes you happy, which in turn makes you more generous. So try it, enjoy it, and benefit from it!

"The meaning of life is to find your gift.
The purpose of life is to give it away."

PABLO PICASSO

THE POWER OF TOUCH: A BIDIRECTIONAL GIFT

Do you cry in airports? I do. If you look around in both arrival and departure terminals, you will see touching (pun intended) displays of emotion. Researchers have documented almost twice as much physical contact between people in airports as in shopping malls. Touch not only conveys emotion more powerfully, but it also drives health and happiness.

Nature has gifted us with five senses, of which *touch* is the first to develop. It plays a critical role in social interactions throughout our lives, and we start experiencing it early. Our first lessons in loving touch start at birth (some say before) with the kissing and cuddling most of us receive from our parents. Touch is associated with pro-social emotions that ensure the well-being of our species. It drives trust and cooperation, and is considered primary societal glue in all primate species. In order to drive nurturing and collaborative behavior, Mother Nature designed rich individual incentives for these tactile instincts. She rewards touch with a host of pleasurable feelings and long-term health, reinforcing our natural urges to touch.

To understand the power of touch, we must follow the biological journey of a peripheral sensory experience from your skin, through sensory nerves, to the pleasure centers in the brain where chemical changes drive the practical benefits associated with touch.

Touch begins in the skin, the largest sensory organ in the body, comprising almost one-fifth of an adult's total weight. There are several different types of sensory receptors in the skin, enabling the owner to perceive a range of sensations. These specialized receptors each detect texture, shape, motion, vibration, pressure, pain, or temperature. When a receptor is stimulated, it rapidly shuttles the message up the sensory nerves to the brain.

The brain then plays an extraordinary role in evaluating the sensation. First, it differentiates between interpersonal (involving someone else), intrapersonal (involving yourself), and passive (involving an inert object) touch. Second, the brain integrates and analyzes all the different sensory messages coming in from your skin at any one moment. Finally, the brain integrates the sensation of touch with other sensory stimuli to draw a final conclusion about the overall experience. For example, your brain will evaluate a firm handshake from a colleague with friendly eyes differently than the same handshake associated with angry eyes.

Once the brain has processed the touch sensations in their full context, it stimulates the release of several powerful hormones. In particular, the body produces dopamine, endorphins, and oxytocin in the presence of favorable touch. These hormones make us *feel* good, encouraging the nurturing and collaborative social interactions that provoke them. These highly desirable feel-good hormones also have important individual health benefits. Empathetic touch has been shown to reduce blood pressure and limit heart rate increases in stressful situations. It reduces stress and anxiety directly, as well as dampening the stress hormone response, which is beneficial because the stress hormone cortisol has a negative impact on immune function over time. Frequent touch, such as that enjoyed in massage therapy, has been demonstrated to strengthen the immune system. Importantly, these benefits are accrued by both those being touched and those doing the touching. Finally, there is good evidence to show that touch reduces pain sensitivity, a phenomenon of both practical and therapeutic value.

There are many experiments that demonstrate the applied benefits of touch. Mothers with postpartum depression are encouraged to massage their babies because it has been shown to improve their own mental states. Also, the amount of tactile affection shown within a long-term relationship proves to be highly correlated with overall relationship success and partner satisfaction. The touch of an empathetic caregiver improves patient adherence to medical advice. Similarly, the kindness shown in an appropriate touch from a salesperson improves consumer trust. Waiters and waitresses who touch their guests (again appropriately) get tipped better. Touch has even been shown to correlate with sporting success—touchy teams win more games!

Some of what we know about the benefits of touch comes from people deprived of tactile stimulation. Some sad early experiments with animals highlighted the physical and emotional retardation that accompany sensory deprivation. More recent research shows that children deprived of tactile support are often below average in both social and cognitive ability in later life. It is no accident that we use the term "tactless" and the phrase "out of touch" to indicate negative states.

There is wide cultural variation in social norms regarding touch. There is strong debate about our right to touch and be touched, especially in the USA today. Fear of litigation and stigmatization, which arose out of good intentions to protect individuals against abusive touch, limits our tactile interactions. Dr. Tiffany Field, Director of the Touch Research Institute in Miami, Florida, claims that we suffer the consequences of this tactile deprivation, something she calls "touch hunger." As a physician, I deeply appreciate the power of my healing hands. This experience and my insight into the underlying science have me strongly supportive of the argument for more rather than less touch, with two precautions. First, mutual consent must prevail; both parties must be entirely comfortable with the physical expression of an emotional message. Second, we must learn to listen with our hands. People quickly show their comfort or discomfort to touch. We must respect their wishes.

Greeting cards often appeal to our emotions through images of happy animals enjoying physical proximity. Cute puppies snuggle together. Loving cats lick and nuzzle their kittens. Mischievous bear cubs wrestle and play together. Monkeys groom each other affectionately. Our affinity for these messages displays our belief in the value of touch, a powerful tool for WHealth Seekers on the road to BodyWHealth.

CONCLUSION

It is clear that for BodyWHealth, we need our emotional brain overflowing with serotonin. Social interaction alone is not enough. We need social *engagement*. We need affirmation and physical contact. More powerfully still, we need to love and to give. We must invest socially and emotionally. When we do this, we are rewarded with both serotonin and BodyWHealth.

Closely linked to social engagement is the other pillar of emotional WHealth, and the seventh Key, living purposefully. In the next chapter, we will look at the science of purposeful living and its profound value in driving WHealth.

KEY #7: LIVE WITH PURPOSE

Embrace a passion bigger than yourself.

In a few remote corners of the globe are populations of people who seem to have cracked the code for longevity. Okinawa, Japan is one of these. Dan Buettner is an explorer who has worked with *National Geographic* and has reported on these age-defying groups, and he refers to their regions as the "Blue Zones" of the world. He explains that there is no word for retirement in the Okinawan language.[61] "Instead, there is one word that imbues your entire life, and that word is 'ikigai.' Roughly translated, it means 'the reason for which you wake up in the morning.'" Makes you think, right?

At the apex of Maslow's hierarchy is the term *self-transcendence*. Heavy words from a learned scholar of human behavior. Self-transcendence is a grand human ideal; it is a sense of belonging to something bigger and more important than ourselves. It is a profoundly motivating and rewarding state of being. Picture some of the world's greatest adventurers and heroes, people who transcend themselves to bring beautiful things to others. The Wright brothers were determined to see humans fly. Mandela, Martin Luther King, Jr., and Gandhi fought to bring social justice to their people. Nobel-winning scientists strive to advance the frontiers of our knowledge. Each are driven by an inspiring purpose, and in their own ways have changed the world as we know it.

Purpose means different things to each one of us. We don't all have to find the way to world peace or invent the next digital era. It could be that purpose for us is simply being the very best contributor we can be at work, helping colleagues to do well and the team to achieve the common goal. It could be that we are focused on having a happy family. We might devote ourselves to the life of a religious or social community. We may have a great artistic talent that we cultivate to bring joy to others.

At its core, purpose implies a sense of intentionality. When we have a goal that is bigger than ourselves that we are passionate about, we have purpose.

That purpose drives us and gives us meaning. When we live purposefully, we know that our daily activities matter. We feel good about our past and enjoy making plans for the future. WHealth Seekers should *embrace a passion bigger than themselves.*

Not surprisingly, Mother Nature has found a way to reward us for purposeful living. For success as a species, we must honor her intention for us to nurture our young and to collaborate with and contribute to our fellow human beings. When we do this, she rewards us with WHealth, and we flourish.

PURPOSE PROLONGS LIFE

Several studies have shown conclusively that purposeful living is associated with longevity. Researchers from Mount Sinai St. Luke's–Roosevelt Hospital[62] aggregated data from a large number of research studies and demonstrated that people with a sense of purpose have a 23 percent lower risk of death from any cause than people without a sense of purpose. That's in the range of the benefits credited to exercise and weight control. Although we can't fully explain this benefit, it is impressive!

The MIDUS (Midlife in the United States) Study[63] evaluated purposefulness in a group of 6,000 American adults, ultimately finding that those with a strong sense of purpose had a 15 percent lower risk of death over the

STUDIES SHOW PURPOSE PROLONGS LIFE

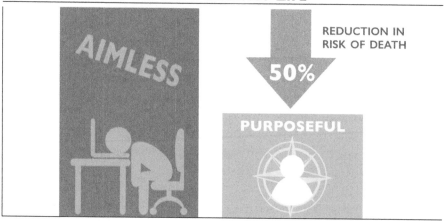

FROM RUSH MEMORY AND AGING PROJECT AND MINORITY AGING RESEARCH STUDY

subsequent fourteen years than their aimless peers. The researchers in that study concluded that purpose provides a "buffer" against death.

On another continent, the English Longitudinal Study of Ageing[64] followed 9,000 people over about a decade. Researchers found that only 9 percent of subjects with a strong sense of purpose died during this period, compared with 29 percent of their peers who reported lower purposefulness.

Scientists from the Rush University Medical Center combined the data from two separate research studies[65]: the Rush Memory and Aging Project, and the Minority Aging Research Study. They tracked over 1,200 community-dwelling older persons for five years, and discovered that those without purpose were almost twice as likely to die than their purposeful peers.

While much of the published research evaluates the risk of death in older populations, where the risk of disconnection and aimlessness is possibly higher, the evidence is nevertheless compelling. I am convinced that the physical impact associated with your choice to be purposeful starts early.

PURPOSE IMPROVES PHYSICAL HEALTH

If you need evidence for the early impact of purpose on your WHealth, let's look at benefits beyond longevity.

For a start, purposeful people care about their health more than their less-purposeful peers.[66] They are more proactive in healthy behaviors, like having regular cholesterol tests, colonoscopies, mammograms, Pap smears, or prostate exams. Not surprisingly, this better preventive health care results in significant reductions in using other health care services, as well as fewer nights spent in the hospital. All because of a sense of purpose!

Perhaps this responsible health screening behavior accounts for all the benefit of a purposeful life? Not so. Other data suggests that this is not the entire story—that something else is going on with a direct biological benefit. Cardiovascular events are reduced by about 20 percent in people who live purposefully.[67] The likelihood of having a stroke was almost halved in one study of purposefulness.[68] These data show us that above and beyond promoting WHealthy behavior, having purpose changes our body chemistry, making us less susceptible to serious diseases.

PURPOSE IMPROVES MENTAL HEALTH

In addition to improving our physical health, purpose also has a profound effect on our mental health, especially as we age. In short, purposefulness protects our brains!

The Rush Memory and Aging Project evaluated almost 1,000 older persons without dementia.[69] Purposefulness reduced the risk of mild cognitive impairment, a serious consequence of aging, by almost 30 percent. More powerfully, over a period of seven years of follow-up, researchers found a highly significant reduction in the risk of developing Alzheimer's disease in purposeful subjects.[70] In fact, their aimless peers were twice as likely to develop Alzheimer's disease! Alzheimer's disease is associated with the accumulation of structural changes in the brain. Although not always associated with Alzheimer's disease, most scientists consider these plaques and tangles to be a sign of the underlying disruption to brain tissue. The Rush study proved that purposefulness protected even those with signs of physical disruption from the cognitive ravages of Alzheimer's disease.[71]

THE BIOLOGY OF PURPOSE

It's not yet entirely clear how purpose rewards us from a biological perspective. On the one hand, it seems logical that purposeful individuals lead healthier lives. When your life has meaning, it is easier to heed the abundant advice that surrounds us all, directing us toward healthy behavior. Life is more valuable when we are purposeful, and we take the big decisions that affect our health more seriously.

There is emerging evidence that purpose also acts directly on the foundational building blocks of BodyWHealth. Like exercise and weight control, purpose appears to have some beneficial impact on our inflammatory balance.[72] Chemicals that suggest domination of the pro-inflammatory cytokine army of decay appear to be reduced in people with greater purpose and devotion to causes bigger than themselves. Purposeful living is also associated with better-quality sleep[73] and better control of stress.[74] It appears that these positive benefits occur deep within our genes.[75] People with a sense of purpose dial down the activity of genes that cause systemic inflammation and compromise the immune system. It is not surprising, then, that purposefulness drives BodyWHealth.

CONCLUSION

When you live with purpose, you improve your physical, mental, and emotional health. You see yourself from a more positive perspective and appreciate that you are valuable. With purpose, you can climb to the highest rung of Maslow's ladder, achieve self-transcendence, and prosper. That is the peak of WHealth.

WHEALTH PLUS

Your two highest priorities to ensure emotional WHealth are to engage socially and to live purposefully. With these guides in place, you unlock the orchards of abundance. The fruits below outline a few of life's greatest riches, exploring their scientific origins and profound value for WHealth Seekers.

THE POWER OF SMILING: THE BEST EXERCISE

You may be wondering why exercise suddenly pops back up in the section on Emotional WHealth. What if I taught you a single exercise that worked more than twenty muscles, and improved your health *and* happiness? What if I told you that you could do it anywhere, anytime, that it wouldn't cost a cent, and that it benefits those around you? What if I told you that those who do it with the greatest intensity are rewarded with the longest lives? And what if I told you that this exercise was to simply smile?

You might be surprised to learn that the face is a highly mobile body part that includes forty-three muscles (depending on how you count them; some are paired). All of these muscles are activated by a single nerve, the *facial nerve*, one of twelve nerves that come directly out of the brain. Scientists refer to these muscles as the "muscles of facial expression" because that is their job. They twist, tweak, and contort our faces so that we can communicate beyond words. We need a spectacular body part to perform this extraordinary, complex role.

In theory, if you were to do the math on the number of unique facial gestures each of us could make, the figure would be an astounding 8.8 trillion! That is 8.8 followed by twelve zeros! With a global population of about 8 billion, this means that I would have over 1,000 unique facial expressions to share with each person on the planet. Or, I could use 300 million new expressions every day of my life. Whew!

In practice, even if our faces could execute all of these gestures, our brains are not big enough to interpret each discrete nuance. Instead, scientists and computers are able to decipher twenty-one unique, consistently differentiable categories of facial gesture.[76] We can break these down further to six major emotions: *happiness, sadness, surprise, fear, anger,* and *disgust.* Some researchers add *contempt* as a seventh. The reason we get twenty-one categories out of these six emotions is that some are compounded. For example, your face can show that you are either happily surprised or sadly surprised. It is this remarkably nuanced communication repertoire that makes our face such a rich communication tool.

Of all these expressions, one stands out as having extraordinary WHealth benefits: the simple smile. There are, of course, a broad variety of real-life smiles: the shy smile, the smug grin, the naughty smirk, the delighted beam, and many more. They are all good for you.

How does this fundamental expression of happiness benefit WHealth Seekers? Let's first start with how it benefits *others.* Smiling is contagious. Research has proven, beyond doubt, that a smile induces others to smile. This is as true with family and friends as it is with perfect strangers. In fact, the power of this life force is so strong that smiling photographs are enough to evoke happiness. This means that each time you smile at somebody else, you give him or her the same benefits that you also enjoy for yourself.

And when you exercise your twenty-plus smiling muscles in beautiful harmony, you benefit personally in six primary ways. First, you experience *better cardiovascular health.* Smiling reduces blood pressure, which contributes to a decrease in heart disease. Second, you experience *reduced stress.* Smiling releases dopamine, endorphins, and the feel-good hormone serotonin, all of which enhance mood and reduce the adverse effects of stress. Unsurprisingly, then, the third benefit of smiling is *enhanced mood.* Independent of the second benefit of reduced stress, the act of smiling makes you happy. Darwin was the first scientist to recognize that "even the simulation of an emotion tends to arouse it in our minds."[77] Modern researchers know this as the *facial feedback hypothesis.* It is much easier to control our muscles than our emotions, so smiling is a simple way to influence our mood and emotions for the better!

The fourth benefit of smiling is *increased attractiveness.* Research has shown many times over that a smiling face is more attractive to others than a non-smiling face. Whether you're trying to find a mate, work well with colleagues, or simply live more easily, smiling works. Smiling's fifth benefit is *better relationships.* People who smile more have more stable and satisfying marriages and long-term relationships. Finally, smiling *improves longevity*. This is the ultimate evidence for the value of smiling. In a landmark study, scientists demonstrated how those who tended to smile lived longer than fake-smilers, who lived longer than non-smilers. Pretty astounding!

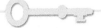

"Sometimes your joy is the source of your smile,
but sometimes your smile can be the source of your joy."

THICH NHAT HANH

THE POWER OF LAUGHTER: A WHEALTHY CONTAGION

Close your eyes and picture a happy gathering. Visualize the faces of friends and family. Close your eyes tighter, squeezing out all other senses except sound. Hear the noises of happiness. I'd be very surprised if laughter wasn't there, possibly even the dominant sound memory. And that's true for good reason; this explicit social expression drives health and happiness.

As we begin to interact with the world as tiny infants, we watch and copy those around us. Before our brain develops the connections that enable speech, we learn to smile and laugh. This is a curious phenomenon that emphasizes the value of that immensely powerful act. You might question why babies would choose to copy something that adults do with much lower frequency than children. Actually, it's not so surprising. Adults laugh far more in the presence of babies than they do elsewhere, underlining laughter's deep association with true happiness.

Laughter is a spontaneous gesture that is triggered unconsciously. Unlike smiling, laughter cannot be forced, making it a hard subject for scientists to study. We know that the average adult laughs seventeen times a day. The vast majority of times, it's not in response to a joke, indicating that it's less an expression of humor than it is an expression of comfort and familiarity (or sometimes nervousness). We laugh much more when we are with other

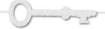

> "When the first baby laughed for the first time, its laugh broke into a thousand pieces, and they all went skipping about, and that was the beginning of fairies."

J.M. BARRIE, IN PETER PAN

people, reinforcing the role of laughter in interpersonal bonding, a profoundly WHealthy engagement.

Only humans laugh, making laughter a precious gift granted us by Mother Nature. The gesture is unique to our species because it involves the three major centers of the brain. Gelotologists (laughter scientists) have identified electrical activity in the cerebral cortex and limbic system during laughter. The chemical response is a reduction of stress hormones. Laughter inhibits the fight and flight response driven by our primitive reptilian brain, with very healthy consequences.

Laughter appears to have several physical benefits, including a decrease in blood pressure, an increase in blood flow, and an increase in oxygenation of the blood. It also recruits activity from the facial, core, and respiratory muscles. It is estimated that a hundred laughs are equivalent to fifteen minutes on an exercise bicycle! Laughter has further been shown to strengthen the immune system. It increases blood cells that are involved with attacking alien cells like foreign pathogens (infections) and cancer. It also increases the cells that are responsible for antibody production. These benefits may all be related to the decrease in stress hormones that is associated with laughter. Unopposed, these stress hormones suppress the immune system, increase blood pressure, and increase the number of platelet cells in the blood (which predisposes us to heart attack and stroke). As with smiling, laughter also releases dopamine, endorphins, and the feel-good hormone serotonin.

Like smiling, laughter is contagious, as anybody who has ever "gotten the giggles" knows. So, when we laugh with friends, we not only benefit personally, but we share that health and happiness with others.

I have often found it sad that we laugh less as adults than we did as children. It seems that once we get "serious" about life, we cannot be seen to be trivial or frivolous. If only we could remember that laughter is a great medicine, and one with no negative side effects. Try it for a few days, and see what happens!

THE POWER OF IMAGINATION: FUEL FOR PURPOSE

What did you pretend to be when you were growing up? A doctor, a nurse, an astronaut, a soldier, a teacher, a dolphin trainer? Personally, I loved being Robin Hood. I have old black-and-white photographs of me dressed in a green outfit, bow and arrow in hand, presumably dispossessing the rich to feed the poor.

In playing these imaginary childhood games, we are actually planting some of the most important seeds of our lives. Freeing our imaginations empowers us to live purposefully, for our imaginations know no bounds.

I often sat watching lion cubs in the wild in my native South Africa. If you've had this privilege, I'm sure that you too were mesmerized by their miniature worlds. They start as cute little balls of fluff that you want to hold and

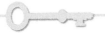

"Imagination is more important than knowledge.
For knowledge is limited to all we now know and
understand, while imagination embraces the entire world,
and all there ever will be to know and understand."

ALBERT EINSTEIN

cuddle. They end up as majestic killers. How is this massive transformation possible? Of course, there is something in their DNA that drives a biological maturation process, but there is more to this mystery. The clue is in watching the play of these furry cubs as they begin to explore their world.

These little creatures engage in robust physical play. Their lives seem to be one long game. They stalk, pounce, chew, bite, ambush, and chase each other continuously. Their comical antics are punctuated only by periods of feeding and sleep. In their little minds, the flicking tail of their mother becomes the prey that will feed their own offspring. A gentle snarl or swipe from a giant maternal paw brings them back to reality. As they stalk their sister, they imagine a juicy fat antelope. As they square up against their brother, bristling and snarling, standing as tall as possible, they imagine themselves defending their pride against competing predators. These imaginary games empower their future purpose.

To understand this, we must return to our knowledge of the neurobiology of the brain. As you probably recall, our giant cerebral cortex differentiates us from other mammals. Mother Nature has given us this center of thought and reason as a powerful tool. It is fully under our control and able to override the other two brain centers: the emotional brain (which drives empathy and love), and the primitive brain (which drives flight and fight survival instincts). A powerful thought or idea that originates in the cerebral cortex, when coupled with a strong desire from the emotional brain, becomes *belief*, which in turn suppresses the negative, protective influence of the primitive brain. *Belief* is the cornerstone of the mansion of success.

Belief in their purpose is why lion cubs play. They are exercising their cognitive brains with the aspirations and ideas of future success. *Belief in their purpose* is why children play. If you carefully peel back the layers of memory, you will realize that you weren't pretending to be a cowboy, but that in your mind, you actually *were* one. You weren't pretending to be a caring teacher educating and nurturing little human beings—you actually *were* one. You weren't pretending to be a doctor saving lives—you actually *were* one. You weren't pretending to explore new frontiers in space as an astronaut—you actually *were* one. That's the power of imagination.

These imaginative games aren't only for cubs and kids. They are the foundation of success for adults, too. Walt Disney could not have built his fantastical entertainment empire without imagination. Steve Jobs could not have built the Apple corporation without first imagining a beautiful, sleek handheld device that would one day connect us intimately and wirelessly with those we love. We would not have put Neil Armstrong on the moon if not for the powerful imagination of early NASA scientists. Every journey starts with a vision, a tiny seed from your cognitive brain that grows in your imagination. Nurtured by desire from your emotional brain, it becomes *belief*, and fuels purposeful success.

Plant those seeds of purpose. Play. Imagine. Dream. *Believe.*

THE POWER OF AWE: A FOUNDATION FOR ENGAGEMENT

When did you last stand in awe? Were you gazing at a pounding ocean? Lying on your back contemplating the night sky and the vastness of the heavens? Watching the poetry of ice-dancing? Enjoying the athleticism and spectacle of the Super Bowl? Listening to your favorite music? Reading about the life and work of a great hero, a social evangelist, or an agent for change?

More importantly, do you remember how you felt? Do you remember the flood of warmth, the deep respect, the feelings of littleness, or perhaps the inspiration?

Awe inspires powerful emotional engagement.[78] Research shows that the sense of humility and comfort we feel when we recognize that we are part of a greater entity, such as nature or humanity, increases both empathy and gratitude. These are powerful pro-social emotions that stimulate social engagement.

So, find your awe. Bathe yourself in it, often. Enjoy it. Share it. Savor it. That's the road to WHealth!

THE POWER OF MUSIC: ENGAGING ALL OF YOU

Music reaches our hearts and minds, plucking chords that resonate deep within our bodies and brains with an impressive range of physical, mental, and emotional benefits. These benefits will aid you in living a socially engaged and purposeful life.

Several intriguing aspects of music make it a multifaceted stimulant, provoking your engagement in a broad range of mental skills. Unlike other mental exercises, music (especially playing an instrument) engages both the left and right brains. Music is full of patterns, both in pitch and in timing, that entertain and stimulate our brains. With its temporal continuity, music can also train the brain to interpret the present in the context of the past and to anticipate the future. This is a key evolutionary advantage that differentiates the human brain from that of other species, and a principle that may underpin a great deal of music's cognitive value—as well as giving us the proper mindset for living purposefully.

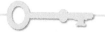

"If music be the food of love, play on..."

DUKE ORSINO IN WILLIAM SHAKESPEARE'S TWELFTH NIGHT

Music has been shown to have a host of physical benefits that enhance BodyWHealth. Exercise is central to WHealth, and music has several beneficial effects on training. Music enhances motivation and reduces perceived exertion. As a result, workout rate and endurance both improve, enabling better-quality workouts.

Soft background music (particularly when paired with dimmed lights) has been shown to reduce food consumption during a meal. Gentle music slows your eating, allowing your fullness cues to trigger earlier in the meal—before you have gorged yourself. Sleep quality can also be improved with music. Studies have shown more rapid sleep onset in participants listening to music, especially infants and young children. Listening to classical music while falling asleep (and I'm sure gentle music of other genres would have the same effect) has been shown to treat insomnia and reduce daytime drowsiness in college students, a benefit easily extrapolated to the rest of us, too.

Cardiovascular health can be directly affected by music, probably through its effect on stress reduction. In one study, thirty minutes of listening to music was shown to reduce blood pressure and heart rate. Another interesting experiment demonstrated enhanced vascular reactivity in the presence of joyful music. This is an important measure of cardiovascular health, although the mechanism causing the benefit is uncertain. Laughter had a positive similar impact, while jarring music that provoked anxiety had the opposite effect.

Several studies have shown the effects of music on immune function, although the overall effect on improving resistance to infection is hard to demonstrate. Researchers speculate that part of the benefit arises from the reduction in cortisol, the stress hormone that dampens immune function. Soothing music has been shown to increase levels of *IgA*, an antibody involved in the first line of defense against infection. Other antibodies in the blood have also been shown to increase after participants listened to as little as fifty minutes of uplifting music. Not only is cortisol reduced and antibody levels increased, but scientists have also reported a reduction in IL6, the pro-inflammatory cytokine that has a strong association with diseases such as heart disease and cancer.

While the physical benefits of listening to music are wonderful, the mental and emotional benefits are even more impressive.

Research has shown that music impacts the levels of several of the brain chemicals that play important roles in mental and emotional health. Listening to joyful music releases dopamine, a feel-good hormone, in the brain. Music also has an effect on serotonin levels, which improves long-term mood regulation, memory, and sleep. The brain releases endorphins when you listen to music you enjoy, independent of genre or tempo. Finally, research has shown that music affects the levels of oxytocin, the love hormone. This hormone is deeply involved in bonding and social recognition. Collectively, these effects explain the profound feelings evoked by music—and all of them improve your sense of self-value, enabling you to live a more socially engaged and purposeful life.

As a result of these chemical responses, music has been shown to relieve *stress* and elevate mood. Calm music has been shown to impact brain waves and induce meditative states that can enhance emotional and mental performance. Other research has shown that music reduces anxiety as effectively as massage. Music has been used to reduce stress and anxiety both pre- and post-operatively.

Many studies have demonstrated enhancements in cognitive function after listening to music. When this benefit was first discovered, it was dubbed the

"Mozart effect" because the first experiment had subjects listening to music composed by Mozart. Subsequent research demonstrated that other music had the same impact, and suggested that it was perhaps the enjoyment of the music, rather than the music itself, that drove the benefit. Several aspects of mental power have been evaluated separately, including reading, spatial reasoning, concentration, and memory. Under the right circumstances, using the right music, all these cognitive functions have been shown to improve. I am particularly interested in the emerging evidence that active engagement in music (that's not just listening, but playing an instrument or singing) may help ward off the mental deterioration associated with aging, and even decrease the risk of dementia. Hopefully, research will clarify this further in the future.

Finally, music has proven useful in the treatment of several disease states.

Music has the ability to relieve depression in some patients. This is true for classical and meditative music especially. Unfortunately, heavy metal music actually makes depression worse.

Music can meaningfully reduce the perceived intensity of pain, especially in geriatric care, intensive care, and palliative medicine. Music not only distracts and relaxes patients, but it also releases endorphins that have benefit in reducing the pain associated with arthritis, surgery, and migraines.

Fascinating research into the use of music in the rehabilitation of brain injuries, such as those experienced after stroke, have shown clear benefit. Music can be used to regain partial or full access to memories. After suffering a stroke, people will often have speech impairments as a result of damage to speech-controlling nerve pathways in the brain. Music evokes "parallel" pathways and may even have the ability to assist in repair of the damaged speech pathways. Making adjacent nerves stronger seems to allow the damaged nerves to recover.

Patients with impaired motor skills, such as those with Parkinson's disease, have also benefited from music therapy. Music can increase their walking speed and help them with the initiation of movement, a classical Parkinson's problem.

Another fruitful area of research has been in the autism spectrum disorders. Music helps with the development of language and motor skills, and activates areas of the brain associated with socialization.

Music engages our entire brain, unlocking unseen links between body, mind, and emotion. It taps into our primal chemistry, unlocking rhythms and melodies buried deep in our genetic origins. Music transcends language and culture, bridging social divide. It evokes passion and pleasure, delivering health and happiness. Savor it, and make it, for WHealth.

THE UNSUNG HEROES:
POSITIVE THINKING AND RESILIENCE

*Tap into the immense power of positive thinking
to unlock resilience.*

Social engagement and purpose are the broad, strong branches of happiness. If you cultivate these, you will build BodyWHealth, enabling you to wander the orchards of emotional WHealth and achieve abundance.

Your journey will be rewarding, I promise. But you may not be surprised that I will infuse a gentle caution: While simple, the path is not always easy. You will meet challenges. Two tools will help you to journey beyond these obstacles, growing from the experience.

We are all equipped with the primal neurobiology for positive thinking, a powerful mindset you can unlock and nurture. Insight and practice will enhance this skill. It will enable resilience, your ability to not only withstand setback, but to triumph over it. This chapter explores the underlying science of both positive thinking and resilience.

FEELING GOOD

If you have ever felt sad, depressed, or anxious, I want you to find and watch the TED talk by Dr. David Burns entitled *Feeling Good*. It's a poignant description of how we can use our cognitive brains to positively affect our moods, and to change lives. Watch all the way to the end.

I started reading and learning about cognitive therapy several years ago. I have always been fascinated by mood. What is it that happens inside our brains that leaves us feeling elated ("on top of the world") or gloomy ("down in the dumps"), and everything in between? More importantly, how can we influence what happens within so that we can spend more time feeling high than low?

A famous American psychiatrist, Aaron Beck, first developed cognitive therapy in the 1960s. His early work defined the cognitive model, which states that thoughts, feelings, and behavior are all connected. His approach can be distilled to three essential insights. First, our thoughts create our moods, and our emotions are the result of the way we interpret the world around us. Second, depression and anxiety are often the result of distorted thoughts. And third and finally, we can be trained to change the way we think, which changes the way we feel.

Cognitive therapy is based on this connectivity between thoughts, feelings, and behavior, and essentially uses the power of cognition (thought) to influence mood and behavior.

Cognitive therapy is the most researched form of psychotherapy and has demonstrated excellent results. A powerful example is in the treatment of depression, where it has been shown to be at least as good as (and many say better than) antidepressant drugs. Depressed thinking is characteristically distorted. Most of us can recall episodes in our lives when we were sad or anxious. We expected the worst. When the sun rose the next morning, and the things we were dreading did not happen, we felt better. And then, if we looked back with bravery and honesty, we might have realized that our fears were exaggerated—we had imagined outcomes that were distorted and unrealistic. Cognitive therapists help depressed patients to identify the thoughts that distress them and to evaluate how realistic they are, before teaching them exercises that modify this distorted thinking. When their thoughts become more realistic, the patients feel better.

Burns, now a world-renowned psychiatrist at Stanford University, led the cognitive therapy revolution in depression. He wrote a pivotal book, also titled *Feeling Good*, which is often used as a therapeutic intervention on its own. The book is given to patients with depression, and it has been shown to improve depression in as many as 70 percent of patients.

This evidence confirms for me the immense power of the cognitive brain on our overall emotional and mental state. If cognitive training is sufficiently influential to resolve severe depression, it suggests that the technique may help us all to become more powerful, happy people. Most of us suffer from self-abusive thoughts. We beat ourselves down, preventing ourselves from having the success we deserve. We tell ourselves we are unworthy. These thoughts are the enemy of BodyWHealth. When we consistently hold thoughts that affirm our worthiness, we unlock BodyWHealth and its abundant riches.

TALKING TO YOURSELF

Here's the problem, though: You now know that at the center of our brain is our primitive brain, charged with the responsibility to protect us. Like a good sentry, it is perpetually on the lookout for trouble. It continues a background chatter that is profoundly negative: "Is anything coming to attack me now? What if somebody is waiting around the next corner to jump on me? Will I be able to run fast enough to escape? Am I brave enough to fight?"

Or, more relevant to today's life: "What happens if I get a horrible disease tomorrow? Should I really hope for health? What if this is not realistic?" "Will my business idea really work? Hasn't somebody else already tried and failed? Why didn't somebody else come up with this idea already? Surely, I'm not the smartest person working in this field?" "What happens if she rejects me? What happens if she already has a boyfriend? How will I survive the embarrassment and rejection?"

This persistent negative questioning, biologically designed with the best of intentions to help you survive, becomes part of your daily mental and emotional psyche. Your emotional brain, sandwiched between your primitive and cognitive brains, is highly vulnerable to this ongoing negative barrage—*unless* your cognitive brain speaks up, loudly and positively. Your emotional brain can only withstand the erosive banter of the primitive brain if your cognitive brain speaks in a louder, more persistent voice, and speaks the language of positivity.

I'm not suggesting that you totally ignore or suppress your inner voice of fear; doing so can lead to greater problems. But it's often a good idea to put doubts and fears aside, agreeing to revisit them once you have managed to shift your overall mindset from negative and fearful to positive and hopeful. I advise anybody who cares to listen not to tackle major life problems at night. I don't mean this literally. I mean that you shouldn't try to make major decisions when your mind is clouded with dark negativity. Wait for the figurative morning, when the sun rises. You're far better equipped to arrive at healthy decisions in the light.

Questions can be very powerful allies. If you're not in a place where you feel robust enough to have your cognitive brain overwhelm your protective primitive brain, then ask powerful questions to overcome the fearful litany. Remember, your cognitive brain is under your voluntary control. Train it to ask questions of your primitive brain. Set your cognitive brain as the challenger, asking your primitive brain to justify the doom and gloom it forecasts.

I also suggest that you respect your primitive brain as you do this, because its negative questions are well intentioned. As you stage the conversation between your cognitive and primitive brains, ensure that the former expresses gratitude for the latter.

The fears we listed previously might provoke cognitive brain responses that go something like this:

Cognitive Brain: "Thank you for keeping me safe! Even when I'm relaxing, you make sure that nobody will ambush me. Is there anything that leads you to believe that somebody is waiting around the next corner? Do you have substantial evidence for this?"

Cognitive Brain: "Thank you for worrying about my health. What if I do not contract a serious disease? What if I really am intended to enjoy robust health?"

Cognitive Brain: "Thank you for urging me to be a little more diligent about my business idea. Did you know that some of the world's greatest inventions were accidents? Did you know that 'ordinary' people change the world all the time?"

Cognitive Brain: "Thank you for protecting my feelings. What if she really does love me, and is as uncertain as I am, and you prevent us from realizing this? And if I'm wrong, are you sure that I won't recover from the embarrassment? Haven't millions of other suitors made the same mistake and gone on to find exquisite happiness in their love lives?"

If there were a quick fix for transforming your brain into this swashbuckling command center that knows no fears, I would write that book and retire. But Mother Nature has structured this intense mental antagonism in a very deliberate way, affording significant power to the primitive brain. Insight, knowledge, and daily practice will enable you to develop the muscles and skills of your cognitive brain, ensuring an enduring, pervasive positivity. It's a habit that will transform your life—and the power to build it is in *your* hands.

POSITIVE THINKING AND PERSPECTIVE

Perspective is a strange phenomenon. By its very definition, it suggests that the same thing appears different depending on your vantage point. The "firm" view we think we have of any object or situation is termed *perception*. This sensory fluidity makes it hard for us to be sure that our reality is valid, and has a profound impact on our sense of self, our happiness, our WHealth— and our purpose.

Happiness is tightly correlated with our sense of personal value. When we give to others, we unleash a chemical cascade in our brains and bodies that includes oxytocin and serotonin. Oxytocin is sometimes referred to as the "love hormone," and its release is clearly associated with positive emotions. Serotonin is the mood chemical, intimately responsible for happiness. The anticipation of giving has similar benefit. When we feel valuable or valued, we have decided that we have something to give to others, something others want. The anticipation of giving, even if it doesn't translate into an act of generosity, makes us feel good.

So, how do we assess whether we are valuable? We tend to look at ourselves in a virtual mirror. Several different perspectives form the reflection we see. The most objective perspectives come from close friends and family in the form of direct feedback. We're sometimes lucky enough to have this. For the most part though, our culture is discrete and sensitive, and for good and bad reasons, we often lack this valuable input. So, we're left to guess what others think of us, using subtle clues like body language as a guide.

The suboptimal nature of these sources leaves us intensely dependent on our own opinion, based on our own perspective. Our close proximity to ourselves makes this a difficult and hazardous exercise. In a well-intentioned effort to impose objectivity on our self-evaluation, we hold ourselves up to others. "Am I more valuable than Mary? Do I give more than Joe? Do more people seek me out than Heather?" These questions are motivated by an earnest effort to assess our value in order to satisfy deep biological instincts that drive happiness.

Stated simply, if we judge that we are valuable relative to Mary, Joe, or Heather, our bodies respond with the production of chemicals that make us feel good. We are happy. If we draw different conclusions, our bodies deny us the chemical reward, and we become sad (or worse).

The problem is that most of us are afraid that we will overestimate our value. We have learned from experience that this is not a pretty sight. So, driven by our protective primitive brains, we invoke conservatism as a default. But this has profound risks, because this instinct leads us toward an error that we scientists refer to as *sampling bias*. Our modesty tricks us into comparing the *best* contributions of Mary, Joe, and Heather against our own *failures*. Other writers have suggested that this is like comparing our own blooper reel against the highlights of other peoples' movies.

How, then, do we ensure that we see ourselves as valuable, enabling us to live purposefully, knowing we are contributing to the world?

First, remember that your view is always only a perspective. Make sure that you formulate an opinion of yourself based on multiple perspectives. Use the insight of friends and family to inform these important opinions. Invite input both actively and through an open and accepting disposition.

Second, avoid sampling bias. Ensure that you are comparing apples with apples. When you reach for the video library, be sure to select your highlight reel—and see your purposeful contributions.

Finally, live with gratitude. Practice this powerful mindset. Keep a gratitude diary. Chronicle the many personal assets and achievements that you are proud of. Actually, as you're doing this, you're writing the script for your highlight reel.

The biological consequences of feeling valuable and purposeful are profound. When your thoughts (in this case about yourself) are enduringly positive, your cognitive brain overrules any fears generated by your conservative, protective primitive brain, and your prevailing perspective is positive and purposeful. This triggers the release of happy hormones, which make you WHealthy.

THE NATURE OF RESILIENCE

I love quotes. They gift you with rapid access to deep pools of rich intellectual and emotional insight in a few well-chosen words. I found an Ernest Hemingway gem in my library of favorites that made me think about the nature of resilience.

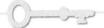

> "The world breaks everyone, and afterward,
> some are strong at the broken places."
>
> ERNEST HEMINGWAY

Actually, I'm still not sure I really like the quote. It has the characteristic Hemingway melancholy, even cynicism. Perhaps it was an inevitable consequence of a life of adventure, perpetually in search of something more. It is clear in his writing that he suffered a persistent sense of loss, and a yearning for reward that seemed to remain beyond his outstretched arms. Nevertheless, Hemingway is one of the great writers, with several titles that are landmarks of twentieth-century literature. His genius was recognized with the Pulitzer Prize for Fiction in 1953 and the Nobel Prize for Literature in 1954.

Here is why I keep the quote in my library of favorites: Without access to our current biological insights, Hemingway seems to understand Mother Nature's intricate design that makes response to injury not only possible, but highly successful. Our fundamental material constituents are in a state of constant flux. Our bodies are a thriving balance of breakdown and reconstruction. We have an ingenious design, where teams of dedicated chemicals and cells destroy the old and broken, while other teams follow them around rebuilding and rejuvenating. Even bone, the strongest of human tissue, is constantly being remodeled, adapting to new stresses to optimize its performance. It is well known that the healing process often leaves injured sites stronger than they were before the insult. I'm sure this is true for our emotional and spiritual existence, too!

I don't like Hemingway's assertion that the world will break everyone. Happy people see a world of opportunity where others see danger. Hemingway's struggle with depression and his ultimate suicide speak to his darker views. But let's assume that as we pursue positive lives of healthy adventure, there is risk of injury and setback. Few could argue against this. In this case,

Hemingway's quote reminds us of the tremendous strength to be gained in healing, both physical and emotional. As in the case of bone, we develop new strength to accommodate new stresses and pressures, and this strength often exceeds anything we had before!

Resilience is a topic of much interest to both social scientists and WHealth Seekers, for good reason. It drives two outcomes we care about: happiness and success. Happy people bounce back with smiles. Successful people "roll with the punches," getting up quickly to continue their journeys. This analogy, originally coined by a great military leader, was subsequently adapted by two famous sporting legends (one living, and one imaginary).

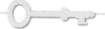

"It's not how many times you get knocked down;
it's how many times you get back up."

COLONEL GEORGE CUSTER

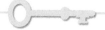

"It's not whether you get knocked down;
it's whether you get back up."

VINCE LOMBARDI

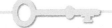

> *"It ain't about how hard you can hit.*
> *It's about how hard you can get hit and keep*
> *moving forward. How much you can take,*
> *and keep moving forward."*
>
> ROCKY BALBOA

Here is the terrifying observation lurking in Hemingway's quote and mirrored in the other three: The power of resilience is not apparent in all people! He alerts us that only *some* appear to respond positively to injury. Only *some* come back stronger. Only *some* get back up. Only *some* keep moving forward. It is probably better to characterize this as a continuum of responsiveness than an all-or-nothing phenomenon. Some seem to wither at the first obstacle. Most survive, moving forward with varying degrees of long-term dysfunction. But there are those few who thrive, coming back stronger, happier, and more determined after a setback.

What drives our ability to respond with resilience? How can we be sure to be in the tiny group who return stronger after injury?

How Can We Achieve Resilience?

Having used a physical analogy, let's follow Hemingway into nature to learn how we can be more resilient.

First, let's understand that resilience itself is a behavior, not an attribute. It's the outcome of a number of mindsets. Like the symptoms of a disease, we're better off understanding the underlying cause. You can't work on your resilience. You can't say to someone, "Be more resilient." It's not something you can just turn on. Instead, we need to look behind the scenes to understand what drives resilience. Then we can find things to work on.

Our psyches are fundamentally biologic in origin and design. They're hard to study directly, so using the construct of our physical body may be helpful (as it was for Hemingway). In our bodies, we have the opposing forces of degeneration and rejuvenation going on all the time. This is no different in our mental and emotional domains. The default is degeneration. If we do nothing else, life breaks us down. So, the first learning is that we must actively drive mental and emotional rejuvenation if we want to be resilient. Stephen Covey, motivational speaker and author, calls this "sharpening the sword."

BodyWHealth teaches that exercise, energy balance, and sleep drive physical rejuvenation at the cellular, chemical, and even genetic levels. What drives psychic rejuvenation, and thus resilience?

First, you can feed the army of good. Just as your physical body has two armies at work, one destroying and one building, so too your mental and emotional being has two armies at work. We must find and feed the mental and emotional "builders" within. Four mindsets favor this balance.

A *neutral emotional response* to setback enables rapid recovery. You won't often find me recommending that you disengage emotionally. Most of the time I advocate strongly for the value of emotional engagement. It has tangible physical benefits that drive WHealth. But think about the way that your body copes with injury. If your immune and inflammatory cells went into mourning when you sustained a minor laceration, complaining that life was miserable and unfair, you might never heal. Instead, without hesitation, your body sends in the cells of rejuvenation to repair and heal your injured tissue. We should emulate this in our lives. Setbacks are just that. Life is full of them. Get over them fast and heal. Like your bones, your mind will remodel to cope with the new stress or circumstances that could otherwise derail you.

Embracing your *vulnerability* can also be a helpful mindset. Some animals have surrounded themselves with hard exoskeletons for protection. Not humans. We have chosen to enjoy the immense benefits of a soft and delicate exterior. Similarly, we're not always right in our attitudes and planning. Things go wrong. That's okay. Be vulnerable. Mistakes and setbacks are loaded with learning. Embrace both, and bounce back stronger.

Yielding to forces greater than you is another helpful mindset. This seems strange advice in a book largely about success and determination. But there are forces in life that are bigger than we are. This may differ over time, and certainly differs between the various facets of our mental and emotional repertoire. I call this the art of *situational yield*. While embracing an overall determination and unwillingness to give up, recognize where victory is critical and where yielding protects you and preserves your strength for more important matters.

Your psyche thrives on *positive thinking*. Feed it. Your cerebral cortex is under your voluntary control and has the ability to overrule both your emotional and primitive reptilian brains. Actively engage in the proliferation of positive thoughts. Social scientists recognize that we learn *helplessness*. There are circumstances that render us impotent. You must learn to recognize, avoid, and even immunize yourself against this destructive tendency.

Finally, *sleep* is the physical mode in which mental and emotional rejuvenation occurs. Many ambitious people believe that they can repair and refuel on the go. Not true. We are built to recover while we sleep, and sleep debt reduces your resilience significantly. While you sleep, you feed and nourish the army of good.

The second method for driving resilience is to build an environment that favors resilience. Recoil requires soft landings and energy. Loving friends and family help with both. There is strong evidence that we have become more fragile and less resilient as we have advanced socially toward more insular, independent lives. We need to actively maintain those close relationships that support and stimulate mental and emotional recoil.

Positivity is mirrored. Surround yourself with people who understand the value of resilience, friends and colleagues who appreciate the value of making mistakes and the power of creativity. Surround yourself with people who give you energy rather than sucking your energy. Incidentally, the best way to ensure this is to be that person, so make sure you give more energy than you consume.

OVERCOMING HELPLESSNESS

It is no accident that the two drivers of emotional health—social engagement and a life of purpose—both involve relationships beyond ourselves. This is where we find strength, beauty, positivity, and resilience. We are the architects of both our internal and external environments. Smart design in both arenas enables resilience, which drives success.

The opposite of resilience is helplessness: the inability or unwillingness to pick yourself up from the floor, dust yourself off, and get on with life after a fall. The great news is that you can immunize yourself against helplessness, increasing your resilience.

Fascinating insights have emerged from social science laboratories over the last two decades, defining helplessness and coming up with strategies to avoid its negative consequences. Martin Seligman is a professor of psychology at the University of Pennsylvania. He is well known to be one of the founders of the Positive Psychology movement. In collaboration with many global thought leaders, he spearheaded our current understanding of helplessness.

Initially in animals, and subsequently in humans, Seligman and colleagues identified a state he termed "learned helplessness."[79] In this condition, the subject acts helplessly under duress. In early experiments, his laboratory dogs (which I'm sure he treated with great kindness) literally lay down in response to what they perceived to be overwhelming circumstances. You can see the close analogy to the pugilist who doesn't get up from the canvas after a big punch, or to the way you feel at the end of a hard day that has tested your resilience.

When he delved further, Seligman found that helplessness is often the result of preceding circumstances in which we are taught that our own efforts are meaningless. Whether at home, or in school, or at work, or all three, when we are taught that our actions are of no consequence, we become helpless. This is learned helplessness. Imagine the young child who tries to win the approval of a parent or teacher by working hard at school. Regardless of his or her efforts, though, the parent or teacher focuses on the questions that the child got wrong, or the talent of the children who got better grades. The child learns that his or her actions (how hard he or she works) have no impact on the desired outcome (affirmation from the parent or teacher). There is grave risk of this young person developing learned helplessness.

Rather than bouncing back after a particularly hard exam, he or she may lie down and give up.

The danger in this situation is that children and young adults are prone to extrapolating their helplessness to other situations. Some personalities, especially those with more pessimistic tendencies, are likely to allow this helplessness, which was specific to their grades, to extend into other functional domains. They begin to feel that their actions are meaningless across a broad range of important areas.

Of course, the opposite is true too. Children who are taught that their actions are meaningful, especially those who are optimistic by nature, grow in confidence and resilience. These are the people who always seem to bounce back quickly from even major setbacks. It is easy to see how this becomes a virtuous cycle, and how resilience becomes a major contributor to success.

Let's return to the helpless for a minute. I'm sure that each and every one of us (at least the honest ones) has felt helpless at some time in some domain of our lives. The good news is that Seligman and his colleagues were not content to rest after discovering helplessness. They also wanted to know if it could be alleviated.

In a fascinating array of experiments, they were able to show that both animals and people could be retrained to believe that their thoughts and actions mattered. Through a variety of techniques that became the foundations of Positive Psychology, these pioneers demonstrated that we could systematically unlearn helplessness.[81] In its place emerged optimism, positivity hopefulness, a belief that life's problems are surmountable, and a resilience that enables newfound success.

And that's not all. The next discovery was thrilling. Seligman and his exceptional team were able to demonstrate that you could teach hopefulness early. By teaching young animals and humans that their actions were meaningful, they were able to build their life-long resilience. Seligman called this phenomenon "immunization" against helplessness. When they encountered unpredicted setbacks later in life, those who had been immunized were more resilient than their peers who had not received this training.

So, what does this mean for you?

If you're seriously debilitated with helplessness or its big brother depression, please look for professional help. In particular, look for someone who understands Positive Psychology and cognitive therapy. These are powerful interventions, and there is every reason to believe that you will get an excellent result.

For all of us, Seligman's findings can serve as a reminder of the power of the cognitive brain. Doubt, fear, pessimism, and helplessness are products of our primitive, reptilian brains. This part of our brain is responsible for protecting us and keeping us safe. It does a great job for the most part, but if we allow it to dominate our lives, we're in trouble. Nature has equipped us with massive cognitive brains, under our voluntary control, which have immense powers over the rest of our brains. We must use our cognitive brains to drive optimism and resilience.

The five steps of cognitive therapy may be useful as you work to develop your own resilience and overcome any helplessness. Understand that we are helpless when we *believe* that our actions are meaningless. Belief is driven by thoughts. In this context, our thoughts are largely negative explanations for our painful experience (being knocked down). You can confront these negative explanations using five steps.

First, you must recognize the automatic negative thoughts, the helpless thoughts, when you meet resistance. Second, you must dispute the negative thoughts using objective arguments. Your explanations about helplessness are seldom correct! Third, replace the helpless thoughts with different explanations. Rather than thinking that you were knocked down because you are weak (and therefore helpless), explain to yourself that your opponent struck a well-timed, powerful blow. This permits you to remain hopeful in your ability.

Fourth, distract yourself from negative thoughts. Recognize when you brood and hold onto helpless explanations. Action is a great distraction. Fifth and finally, over time, with patience and diligence, you will recognize the common negative assumptions you hold that precipitate helplessness. For example, if you often feel helplessly unloved, it may be because you believe that everybody should love you. When a single person doesn't, or makes a single but powerful unloving statement, you collapse helplessly. Challenge your assumption that *everyone* should *always* love you.

Remember as you're combatting your own helplessness and building your resilience to scrutinize your conduct with your children, your students (if you're a teacher), and your subordinates (if you're a boss). You're in a powerful position to evoke either hope or futility. Especially with children, you *will* influence their long-term resilience by your actions. Choose them wisely.

And here's a bonus reward for your efforts: There is ample scientific evidence that optimism improves health and drives longevity, even strengthening your body against some of our greatest medical fears, like cancer. How's that for an incentive?

CONCLUSION

Positive thinking and resilience are powerful tools to combat the negative influence of the sadness, depression, and anxiety with which we all struggle at some point, and to overcome the challenges we will meet on the pathway to abundance. Use the immense power of your cognitive brain to overcome the fear propagated by your primitive brain, allowing your positivity and resilience to shine through.

In Greek mythology, a magical creature symbolizes human resilience. The phoenix is an eternal bird that dies in a bright flash of flames, only to be reborn out of the ashes. May the recurrent rejuvenation of this magical creature inspire you toward the physical, mental, and emotional resilience and positivity required to attain abundant WHealth.

YOUR PRESCRIPTION FOR WHEALTH

Now you understand some of the neuroscience behind happiness, and how the things you do to engage socially and live purposefully drive that happiness.

I wrote about the role of serotonin in the emotional brain, which is the part of the mammalian brain that took us past simple survival instinct and gave us love. In truth, the emotional brain is more important for the behavior it drives than the feeling it gives us. The purpose of the emotional brain is to allow us to care for children (and family) and collaborate with other people. So, if you want to boost your serotonin levels, then love your children and engage purposefully with others—whether just for fun, in community service, or at work.

There are many quick-fix myths about serotonin, the happiness hormone. Here are some triggers that are scientifically proven to increase its levels in your brain; try them.

First, *physical contact* is a powerful serotonin trigger. Snuggling, cuddling, massage, and back rubs all boost serotonin levels (and have been shown to reduce the stress hormone cortisol, too).

Exercise boosts tryptophan, a precursor of serotonin, as well as endorphins that also enhance mood. When you work out with a friend or loved one, the added social engagement benefits you all the more.

Light triggers serotonin. Your serotonin levels are higher in summer, and higher on longer days, so bathe your life with sunlight during the daytime hours—and bring your family outside with you so that you can all benefit.

Eat serotonin-favorable *foods* like dark chocolate and omega-3 fatty acids, and drink red wine, which contains resveratrol that boosts both serotonin and endorphins. Share mealtimes with friends or family to increase the benefit. Limit your caffeine intake because it opposes serotonin.

Finally, find ways to *de-stress*. There is some evidence that long-term stress erodes your serotonin levels, so for many reasons, find ways to avoid it. And remember that engaging with other people is proven to be a powerful reducer of stress.

I hope that by now you are leaping out of your seat with the desire to remind me that I have left out the most important driver of happiness: you and your immense mental capabilities! Your huge cerebral cortex has equipped you, above all other creatures on this planet, to control your own emotional destiny, social engagement, and purpose. It's all in *your* hands!

Simple Recommendations for Unlocking Emotional WHealth

1. *Engage.* The fabric of your own life must merge with the lives of others. Share their journeys. Help them carry burdens. Celebrate their victories.

2. *Love, more than you think is possible.* Remember that love combats fear.

3. *Give, more than you think is reasonable.* Make the value you exude and share with the world appreciably less than what you take from it. Make sure that people are better off when you leave than when you arrived.

4. *Touch, often.* Offer warm, loving (but appropriate!) touches to everyone you can.

5. *Smile, often.* Look people in the eye and share joy and kindness. Speak to others face to face, using video-chat apps if necessary rather than the telephone. Use emoticons when you text.

6. *Laugh, often.* Laugh out loud. Laugh alone. Laugh with others. Laugh *with* people, not *at* them.

7. *Surround yourself with positive, resilient people.* The more, the merrier, literally!

8. *Trust the people around you.* Seek and embrace the benefits of social engagement and friendship. Strangers are friendships that haven't happened yet.

9. *Volunteer.* Give your time to others, detour from your route to help others, and work for the success of others.

10. *Live with purpose.* You are part of something bigger than you that drives and inspires you—live that way!

11. *Live on purpose.* Be proactive more than reactive. Work deliberately to achieve your goals and manage your resources. Run your life and manage your calendar, rather than having your life and calendar running you.

12. *Believe that life is easy.* With this perspective, obstacles become challenges. You become the master of your own destiny. The journey becomes fun!

13. *Focus on things that bring you joy.* Understand what gives you meaning and find ways to build it into your life.

14. *Use positive, purposeful words.* Complaints, negative reflections on the past, and speculation about the activities of others are energy traps. Gossip is toxic. Direct your energy forward, moving positively toward your purpose.

15. *Concentrate on what's right in this world.* Positive conclusions about the world drive your energy and optimism.

16. *Avoid energy drains.* Move quickly away from activities and people that induce negativity, and divert your energy to uplifting activities and people.

17. *Appreciate your gifts.* Recognize your unique strengths and talents, and be grateful for them. Apply them deliberately to advance your journey, to help those around you, and to make a difference.

18. *Don't compare yourself to others.* Be comfortable in your *own* skin. Know that you have something unique to offer the world.

19. *Don't harbor jealousy.* Invest time celebrating rather than mourning the success of others.

20. *Be mindful.* Live in the present. Be thankful for your past, without regrets. Be hopeful and excited for the future; you may be nervous, but don't be fearful of what lies on the journey ahead of you. While appreciating every current moment, know that your best day is ahead of you still.

21. *Consider your future with calm and confidence.* Rather than picturing the few things that can go wrong, spend time imagining success in exquisite detail. Belief fuels success.

22. *Make time for awe.* Find your awe, whether in music, art, nature, sport, or adventure. Then indulge in it.

23. *Empower your cognitive brain.* Remember that it can overcome any fear your primitive brain throws at you if you give it the chance. Practice using it, building its positive muscles until overcoming your fears is a reflex.

24. *Respect your primitive brain.* Remember that it's there to protect you. Appreciate how it ensures your safety, and learn to discern when it's alerting you to real threats.

25. *Stage productive conversations.* Use your cognitive brain to respectfully disagree with your primitive brain.

26. *Foster a neutral emotional response to setbacks.* Bad things happen. Get over it. Build forward positively.

27. *Embrace vulnerability.* In gentleness is awareness and strength.

28. *Yield (selectively) to forces greater than you.* The river wins when it flows around the big boulders, bringing life and energy downstream.

29. *Avoid rigidly controlling your life.* Life happens. Success, happiness, and purpose come from adapting your plans and seizing the opportunities presented by change.

30. *Recognize and dispute automatic negative thoughts.* Be mindful of your internal discussion. Reject automated doubt and fear.

31. *Embrace and foster optimism.* Your mental and emotional response to events is critical. Practice optimism.

32. **Be thankful.** Gratitude for who you are and what you can contribute is a powerful, purposeful force.

33. **Believe.** Trust your abilities. Know that you can accomplish anything you put your mind to.

34. **Expect WHealth.** It's in *your* hands!

CONCLUSION

Investing socially and living purposefully are the final two Keys, which guide your journey to unlocking emotional WHealth. Once you have implemented them on your life, all that remains is for you to reach out and grasp your prosperity. Do so with gratitude!

THE ROAD TO EMOTIONAL WHEALTH

Have fun.

I conclude every article and message with that same simple salute. If you're signed up for my newsletter, you'll see that I sign off each week with the same words. I'm an executive life coach who helps clients achieve BodyWHealth. Many come to me with substantial burdens. Yet I still say goodbye to everybody in the same way: "Have fun!"

Fun is contagious good health for you and for everyone around you. Fun is good for you, even if you have serious physical, mental, or emotional challenges—perhaps I should say *especially* if you have major challenges.

Fun is an attitude. It's a physical process that starts deep in your brain. From there, it ignites several important chemical and hormonal pathways. It results in certain characteristics: smiling, laughing, sparkling eyes, relaxed shoulders, and an easy gait. When you have fun, you reach out and touch other lives. All of these actions both spread goodwill and reward the giver. It is a powerful virtuous cycle.

When you have fun, your body releases hormones that elevate your mood. The act of smiling alone, even if you aren't truly enjoying yourself, releases the feel-good hormone serotonin, which directly elevates your mood and indirectly counters the negative impact of stress. Laughter adds more benefits, like improved cardiovascular health, longer life, and a stronger immune system.

When you're having fun, you reach out more to others, physically and socially. Both bring health benefits. Affectionate physical contact stimulates the release of several powerful hormones. Dopamine, endorphins, and oxytocin all work directly to elevate mood while reducing stress and anxiety. They have a beneficial effect on blood pressure, heart health, and immune strength. Reaching out socially is also a powerful driver of emotional health. This is more pronounced when you engage with others, rather than simply connecting with them. When you have fun, you take the social interaction beyond a superficial connection into the territory of deep engagement. Abundant rewards follow.

When I suggest to people that they "have fun," it implies that they have active control over their dispositions. This is true. We have voluntary control over our thoughts. We can lead our brains toward positive thinking. The cognitive brain then co-opts the emotional brain, and we convert thoughts of fun into a desire for fun. Together, the cognitive and emotional brains override any reservations harbored in the protective and conservative primitive brain. The result is that you do actually have fun! So, even if you don't feel in the mood for fun—and perhaps haven't felt in the mood for some time—you are still able to change your central wiring in a positive way. If you do this often enough, for long enough, fun becomes a healthy habit. As I've said before, any behavior that you deliberately sustain for forty-two days becomes entrenched. Try entrenching fun!

Finally, remember to be thankful for fun. Appreciation is an immensely powerful mindset. It not only reinforces the virtuous cycle with a positive feedback loop, but it becomes explicit to the world in the form of gratitude, a potent force for good in your life and in the world around you.

When I say that tiny little phrase "have fun," I hope you understand that it's not a trivial, throwaway expression. Instead, it's a meaningful plea for you to manifest the cognitive and emotional state that will bring light, health, and happiness into your own life, and the many lives that you touch.

CONCLUSION

Now you have all the tools you need for WHealth. You are well equipped to build upon the physical foundation you've constructed with the first three Keys to physical WHealth. You are empowered to embrace the enabling mindsets, and to use the two Keys that will unlock emotional WHealth.

Health, happiness, and prosperity await you. Go get them—you have the Keys; the power is in *your* hands!

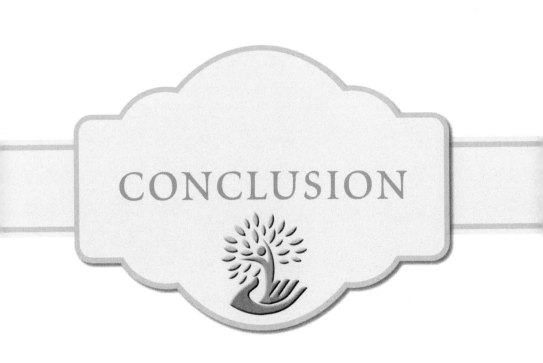

CONCLUSION

My road to BodyWHealth started a long time ago. I was a fresh-faced high school student. I sat waiting to be interviewed for a place at a prestigious medical school. I was excited to start my adult journey. Armed with optimism, enthusiasm, and little else, I looked at the panel of senior medical interviewers in gray suits and white coats. A friendly man who turned out to be the dean of the medical school started. "Why do you want to be a doctor?" Without hesitation, I responded, "I want to help people." In that one sentence, I had said everything.

I have enjoyed a fantastic career and have helped many people in many different roles. I'm not finished yet. Far from it. In fact, in many ways, I'm only just beginning. You see, I now know something about life, and science and medicine, that can't be learned from a book. The taste of BodyWHealth is a powerful insight that can only be experienced firsthand.

BodyWHealth is a state of profound physical and emotional fulfillment. It is a state of deep contentment. It is more valuable than health or wealth alone. BodyWHealth is an investment strategy based on solid scientific principals that optimize your biology and reward you with abundant riches, including health, happiness, and prosperity.

I'm now on a mission to share BodyWHealth with everyone I can. I hope that my insight and experiences can help many more people. I have friends, family, and colleagues who deserve to enjoy BodyWHealth. I have former patients and current clients who deserve to enjoy BodyWHealth. And there are millions of people whom I haven't met yet who deserve to enjoy BodyWHealth, too.

BodyWHealth is a journey. I will be successful if I help only one person—you—to take that path. I am honored that you have chosen to join me!

BodyWHealth: My Journey

My personal BodyWHealth journey started several years ago, when I was in my mid-forties. Actually, I had made a few prior attempts at WHealth, each of which failed. Despite my deep personal and professional understanding of health and happiness, I was lost. I had ignored the foundations of WHealth and was paying the price.

My own path to BodyWHealth started with one step, the same way any journey starts. Intuitively, I knew I had to walk rather than run. So I started stepping, slowly at first. As my bones, ligaments, and tendons grew stronger, I increased my pace and distance until I was achieving 10,000 steps on at least five days of each week. As I built my exercise base, I started to reverse the inflammatory imbalance I had allowed to undermine my health. Sustained exercise supported the enduring resurgence of my anti-inflammatory cytokines. I slowly returned my physiology to its premodern balance. Biology smiled on me.

I started to count the calories I was eating and burning. I made sure that I ate fewer than I burned, aiming for a negative balance of between 300 and 500 calories per day. Over time, slowly but surely, I drained the fat stores that had become the toxic training grounds of my pro-inflammatory armies. And I also started looking and feeling really good!

I made every effort to get a good night's sleep. I knew how this restorative physical and mental window was critical to my ability to continue my hard work.

I realized that excuses would destroy my efforts, and I chose a hard stance. I started my journey in the early part of a very cold, snowy winter. I put on layers of clothing, hats, and gloves, and went outdoors. On a few occasions, my face was almost too cold to continue, and it ached when I came inside afterward. But I was determined to succeed; no excuses!

I did this first for seven days, then for seven weeks, and then for seven months. I rewarded myself with a special prize at each of these major milestones. I knew that the first week would be the toughest; that forty-two days would establish healthy habits; and that after an additional seven months I would have transformed my life. It worked.

I reached a dramatic tipping point one evening. I was struggling with poisonous thoughts of loathing for the body I was trying to escape. I knew what I wanted...no, what I *desired*. But it remained elusive until I stood in front of the mirror, and suddenly, almost by accident, I had a massive mindset shift. I saw myself as a young, healthy, fit athlete. I *believed*. My fate was sealed. The journey took on new vigor. I started to live and act like a young, healthy, fit athlete again, and I became one!

Most people regard this elusive state as unachievable. They see it like confidence or wealth, something reserved for the elite or the very lucky. The powerful truth is that BodyWHealth is within everyone's reach! And *belief* is fundamental to securing it. When we truly believe that we can achieve BodyWHealth, we do.

Now, don't get me wrong. I don't think I'm superhuman. I know that things can still go wrong with my health. I must continue to be vigilant, even as I perpetuate my new WHealth. I still need my doctors; my efforts are in addition to theirs. I still need my cholesterol medication, because there are biological disruptions that many of us have that are beyond this simple fix. I'm delighted that I can live as my ancestors did, but surrounded by the most advanced medical knowledge and technology of today.

At some point on my journey, I crossed an invisible threshold. I attained BodyWHealth. I can't tell you where or when it happened. I just started to feel different. I had suppressed the inflammatory fires that promote disease and degeneration. I had bolstered the anti-inflammatory forces that resist decay, retard aging, and promote rejuvenation. I had rebuilt the physical foundations of WHealth, and I knew it.

The best was still ahead. As I worked on my health, I stumbled upon happiness. I unlocked well-hidden links between body, and mind, and emotion. Having seen me honor my biological design, Mother Nature smiled on me, rewarding me with emotional WHealth.

I now know that happiness is a physical phenomenon. Simple BodyWHealth interventions, well within my control, primed my feel-good chemistry, unlocking internal treasures. I know that social engagement and a sense of purpose are paramount in delivering happiness. I know that the power of loving, giving, touching, laughter, awe, and imagination are gifts, and that mindfulness and gratitude are formidable forces. I know that these all have their origin in our biology, and that in return, they drive physical and emotional WHealth. This is true BodyWHealth.

Finally, I understand that BodyWHealth is both the destination and the journey. I'm delighted that I have so much more to learn and enjoy. Abundance is boundless. I'm happy that I will continue to grow in WHealth for the rest of my life!

BodyWHealth: The World's Journey

As a species, we're on a journey too.

Our ancestors were gifted a biology that equipped them perfectly for a life of physical toil and danger. We have rapidly evolved our technological and societal context. Today, we are less dependent on physical exertion and less vulnerable to acute dangers like predation. There is absolutely no way our biology could adapt at the same speed as our society, and we now pay a handsome price for that truth.

In many parts of the world, we are no longer members of subsistence economies. We have bought ourselves the luxury, free from toil and danger, to focus on emotional WHealth. Ironically, our circumstances have made it too easy to neglect our physical foundation, compromising our ability to build the substantial superstructure of emotional WHealth. We are poor in our richness.

In other parts of the world, a subsistence economy, poverty, and a more physical existence have protected us from the epidemic of degenerative disease that decimates more "developed" society. Infection, violence, and even starvation sadly ravage these parts of the globe. Ironically, in the absence of financial wealth and the presence of a more natural physical existence, many of these people are able to focus on building physical WHealth in a way that escapes us in wealthier corners of the globe.

But for all the world's people, the same pervasive truth exists: There is a WHealth that is greater than either health or wealth alone. The path to this WHealth is through the Body. This is BodyWHealth.

I'm excited for the future of our species. With wisdom and insight, we can restore a biological balance that many of us have lost. We can embrace the wave of technological development that is now focused more than ever on personal health and happiness. We will see more software, hardware, and apps that focus on physical, mental, and emotional health developed over the next ten years than we have seen in all the technology-driven decades before. We will co-opt our advanced technical abilities to preserve a part of history that we have almost lost.

The road to BodyWHealth starts, as its name suggests, within each of our bodies. By understanding and investing in our biology, we optimize our collective health. When we are healthy, we provide the physical and chemical foundations for collective happiness. I can only imagine the far-reaching consequences of global WHealth.

BodyWHealth: Your Journey

This brings me to *your* journey, the most important of all.

I hope that this book has brought you insight and inspiration in equal volumes. I hope that every one of you enjoys a transformative experience in some aspect of your life.

If you're early in your journey, I hope that you will embrace the first five Keys. They're simple, although not always easy. They're designed to help you to rebuild your physical foundation, to stop decay, and to restore health and youth. I know that they work.

If you're already on your journey, perhaps you've tasted WHealth. I hope that you're inspired to continue your personal efforts. I hope that insight into some of the biology behind emotional WHealth encourages you to explore it further. I hope that you're able to embrace the sixth and seventh Keys. I hope that insight into your tiered brain, and the primitive survivalist within us all, enables you to understand and manage your happiness better. I hope that you will strive to master the power of the emotional and cognitive brains in all that you do, driving personal and societal success. I hope that the explanations and insights you derive from these pages enable you to inspire others. In giving, you will receive more.

I hope that every one of you will join the BodyWHealth community, especially through our online portal at www.BodyWHealth.org. Not only will you benefit as a WHealth Seeker, but you can also use the site as a forum to help others who are searching for BodyWHealth. Thank you for your advocacy and support. We have work to do, and it's only just beginning!

It's time now for you to get on with your journey, and me to get on with mine. I am honored to have traveled this short distance with you. I look forward to meeting you on the great road of life, to sharing BodyWHealth stories and insights, and to hearing your BodyWHealth anecdotes and successes.

I look forward to sharing in health, happiness, and prosperity with you.

Have fun,

Roddy

SEVEN KEYS TO UNLOCK WHEALTH

 Step Up

Walk 10,000 steps on at least five days each week.

 Count Calories

Count calories to balance your energy.

 Sleep Right

Cultivate sleep for peak performance.

 Conquer Excuses

Make a commitment that leaves no space for excuses.

 BELIEVE

Believe to achieve.

 Invest Socially

Engage abundantly in your relationships.

Live with Purpose

Embrace a passion bigger than yourself.

ADDITIONAL READING RECOMMENDATIONS

Better Than Before, Gretchen Rubin

Feeling Good: The New Mood Therapy, David D. Burns

Flourish: A Visionary New Understanding of Happiness and Well-being, Martin E. P. Seligman

The Go-Giver: A Little Story About a Powerful Business Idea, Bob Burg and John David Mann

Learned Optimism: How to Change Your Mind and Your Life, Martin E. P. Seligman

The Paradox of Generosity: Giving We Receive, Grasping We Lose, Christian Smith and Hilary Davidson

The Power of Habit: Why We Do What We Do in Life and Business, Charles Duhigg

The Promise of Sleep: A Pioneer in Sleep Medicine Explores the Vital Connection Between Health, Happiness, and a Good Night's Sleep, William C. Dement

The Secret, Rhonda Byrne

Thrive: The Third Metric to Redefining Success and Creating a Life of Well-Being, Wisdom, and Wonder, Arianna Huffington

Triumphs of Experience: The Men of the Harvard Grant Study, George E. Vaillant

Whale Done!: The Power of Positive Relationships, Kenneth Blanchard, PhD, Thad Lacinak, Chuck Tompkins, and Jim Ballard

Younger Next Year: Live Strong, Fit, and Sexy—Until You're 80 and Beyond, Chris Crowley and Henry S. Lodge, MD

GLOSSARY

5-hydroxytryptamine (5-HT): The scientific name for serotonin, a chemical that enables the transmission of messages between nerves (also known as a neurotransmitter) that has been shown to be central to feelings of well-being and happiness.

Adenosine: A molecule that is a building block of our genetic material (both DNA and RNA). It plays a critical role in energy metabolism, sleep, and arousal.

Adipocytes: Fat cells whose primary role is storage of energy.

Adrenal glands: Small organs located near the kidneys that secrete several hormones, such as adrenaline and cortisol. The adrenal glands work together with other organs, including brain centers, to regulate our response to stress, the immune system, energy balance, and mood.

Adrenaline: Also known as epinephrine, a hormone and neurotransmitter that is best known for its role in the body's fight or flight response.

Aerobic exercise: Low-intensity physical exercise that relies primarily on an energy-generating process that burns oxygen for fuel; it can usually be sustained for long periods of time.

Anti-inflammatory cytokines: Small proteins that suppress the inflammatory and immune systems.

Antibody: A large protein that neutralizes invading pathogens, such as bacteria and viruses, as part of our overall immune system.

Antioxidants: Molecules that prevent the chemical degradation of other molecules (a process known as oxidation), which would otherwise result in the production of harmful free radicals.

Atherosclerotic disease: Disease, especially of the heart, brain, and kidneys, that is characterized by thickening and loss of elasticity (hardening) of our arteries, caused by inflammation of fatty deposits in the walls of the arteries.

Autosuggestion: A process in which repeated verbal messages result in a predictable outcome; e.g., if you tell yourself you are tired, you will feel tired.

Basal Metabolic Rate (BMR): The amount of energy expended by the body at rest.

Belief: Deep faith in a current or future state that compels appropriate action and makes success inevitable.

Bipedal primates: Primates that walk upright on two legs.

Brain Plasticity Theory: The belief that the brain is not a static organ, but has the capacity to make significant functional shifts in response to changes in experience and needs.

Brain stem: The central trunk of the brain, which regulates basic functions essential to survival, such as breathing, heart rate, and consciousness (including sleep).

Calorimeter: A scientific instrument used to measure the heat given off by chemical reactions, such as the burning of food fuel.

Cerebral cortex: The outer layer of the mammalian brain (the gray matter) that is responsible for thought, reason, memory, awareness, and language.

Chronic inflammatory overload: Long-term disruption in the inflammatory balance, favoring excessive inflammation.

Circadian rhythm: Any biological process, such as the sleep-wake cycle, that occurs repetitively and predictably within a twenty-four-hour period.

Cognitive behavioral therapy: A form of psychotherapy that was originally designed to treat depression but that is now recognized to have far wider utility; a therapy that alters behavior by shifting unhelpful thinking.

Cognitive brain: The centers of the brain responsible for cognition (thought and reason); loosely centered in the cerebral cortex.

Comfort eating: Food-related behavior that is designed to satisfy an emotional need (such as happiness) rather than a physical need (such as hunger).

Cortisol: A hormone produced by the adrenal glands that plays an important role in the body's response to stress and the control of blood sugar levels.

Cytokines: A large group of small proteins that play an important role in communication between cells, especially those involved with inflammation and the immune system.

Desire: A longing or craving for something that brings satisfaction or enjoyment.

Distress: A state of complete or partial dysfunction as a result of extreme or prolonged stress.

Dopamine: A neurotransmitter that plays an important role in the brain in regulating reward-motivated behavior, in addition to several other functions beyond the nervous system.

Dorsal ganglia: A cluster of sensory nerve cell bodies located close to the spinal cord.

Emotional brain: The centers of the brain (loosely equivalent to the limbic system) that are responsible for mood and instinctive behavior such as nurturing and procreation.

Emotional processing theory: The concept that dreams help us to process complex emotions.

Endorphins: A family of proteins, synthesized by the human body, that interacts with receptors in the brain to produce morphine-like effects of euphoria and lessened pain.

Energy: The force that enables movement or bodily function. Our body consumes energy-rich products and converts them into storable, transportable chemical bonds, such as those in glucose and fat. The combustion of these products, usually in the presence of oxygen, releases energy to fuel biological activity.

Energy balance: The equilibrium that exists between energy ingested (in food) and energy used to drive bodily function and activity.

Energy consumption of activity: The portion of energy burned each day to fuel movement, including exercise.

Eukaryote: An organism that is comprised of cells that each have their genetic material packaged into a single, membrane-bound nucleus; they also have specialized organelles in the cell cytoplasm (the liquid internal environment of the cell) and an elaborate process for multiplication.

Facial feedback hypothesis: A theory that states that our emotions are influenced by facial movements.

Ghrelin: A hormone, also known as the hunger hormone, that is produced in cells located in the intestines and regulates appetite and energy metabolism.

Glucose: The molecular form of sugar that carries and stores energy in the human body.

Glutamate: A common form of glutamic acid, one of the amino acids (building blocks of protein) that is involved in healthy nerve function.

Glutamine: An amino acid (protein building block), related to glutamate, found circulating free in the blood and involved in protein metabolism.

Glycogen: The principal storage form of glucose, found mainly in the liver and muscle tissue.

Inflammatory response: The body's complex response to injury from many different causes, including trauma, pathogenic invasion, and heat injury.

Inflammatory system: The full complement of chemicals, hormones, and cells that react to injury.

Insulin: A hormone produced by the pancreas that regulates the metabolism of glucose and fats.

Interleukins: A family of small proteins (also known as cytokines) that are involved in communication between cells and play a pivotal role in the regulation of our inflammatory and immune systems.

Leptin: Also known as the satiety hormone, a hormone made in fat cells that regulates energy balance by suppressing hunger.

Limbic system: A complex system of nerve centers and networks in the brain, located under the cerebral cortex, that is concerned with mood (including fear and pleasure) and instinct (such as nurturing and procreation behavior).

Melatonin: A hormone involved in synchronizing our metabolism, especially sleep, with the variations of light and dark through the twenty-four-hour day.

Metabolism: The sum of all the chemical processes occurring in the body during any specific time period.

Metabolic disease: Disruption of the chemical processes involved in living, especially those relating to energy balance.

Metabolic syndrome: A disorder of energy utilization and storage that produces a complex clustering of medical conditions that include (abdominal) obesity, elevated blood pressure, elevated blood sugar (glucose), elevated blood triglycerides (fat), and abnormally low levels of high-density lipoprotein (HDL; the "good cholesterol") in the blood; some consider this to be a precursor to type 2 diabetes.

Metabolic rate: The total amount of energy expended to sustain bodily function.

Mitochondria: Cellular organelles that host the important function of cellular respiration (the production of energy) in our bodies.

Neurotransmitter: A chemical substance that transfers messages between nerves or from nerves to other tissue, such as muscles or glands.

Opioid system: The integrated system that includes the opioid (morphine-like) proteins and their receptors, which control reward, addiction, and pain.

Overtrain: The point where performance begins to plateau and then drop as training load exceeds the body's capacity for recovery.

Oxidative free radicals: Also known as antioxidants, these chemicals block the activity of free radicals (naturally formed byproducts of metabolism), which are highly damaging to healthy cells.

Oxytocin: A hormone produced in the mammalian brain that plays a role in bonding, intimacy, and sexual reproduction, in addition to its primary role in stimulating breast milk secretion after childbirth.

Parasympathetic nervous system: Regulates the body's unconscious actions, such as digestion and sexual arousal, during rest.

Pedometer: An instrument that records the number of steps taken by the wearer.

Primitive reptilian brain: The primitive centers of the brain that are common to all reptiles and mammals and are responsible for our most primitive coping functions, such as danger avoidance, territoriality, and other rituals and behaviors that ensure survival.

Pro-inflammatory cytokines: Small proteins that stimulate the inflammatory and immune systems.

Pro-social behavior: Voluntary actions and behavior designed to help other people or society as a whole.

Prokaryotes: Organisms like bacteria and algae that have their genetic material distributed throughout their cellular cytoplasm (fluid in the cell).

Rapid Eye Movement (REM) sleep: The unique sleep phase characterized by random eye movements, low muscle tone, and vivid dreams.

Serotonin: A chemical that enables the transmission of messages between nerves and has been shown to be central to feelings of well-being and happiness.

Sleep cycles: Recurring patterns of consciousness seen in healthy sleep.

Sleep debt: The difference between the amount of sleep you should get and the amount of sleep you actually get.

Slow-wave sleep: The deepest level of sleep, also known as stage 3 sleep, characterized by slow waves of electrical activity in the brain.

Sympathetic nervous system: Regulates the body's unconscious actions, especially the fight and flight response, during activity.

Systemic inflammatory overload: My own term for the inflammatory imbalance that results in the expression of systemic disease (as opposed to localized disease), such as atherosclerosis, diabetes, some of the neurodegenerative conditions, and certain cancers.

Telomere: A section of DNA at each end of a chromosome (an organized string of genetic material), which protects the chromosome from deterioration.

Testosterone: A hormone primarily secreted by testes in men, and to a lesser extent by ovaries in women and adrenal glands in both sexes, that is responsible for the production of male sex organs and secondary sex characteristics like muscle mass and body hair.

Thermic effect of food: The amount of energy burned by our bodies during the processing (digestion and storage) of food.

Threat simulation theory of dreams: The theory that we prepare to cope with dangerous real-life events by rehearsing threatening scenarios in our dreams.

Tonic immobility reflex: The deceptive action taken by certain animals that feign death to escape danger.

Visceral body fat: Fat stores that are located around and between our internal organs in the abdominal cavity.

NOTES

1   "Sedentary Behaviour and Life Expectancy in the USA: a Cause-deleted Life Table Analysis -- Katzmarzyk and Lee 2 (4) -- BMJ Open." BMJ Open - BMJ Journals. Accessed October 29, 2015. http://bmjopen.bmj.com/content/2/4/e000828.full.

2   "Physical Activity | DNPAO | CDC." Centers for Disease Control and Prevention. Accessed October 29, 2015. http://www.cdc.gov/physicalactivity/index.html.

3   "Quantity and Quality of Exercise for Developing and Maintaining Cardiorespiratory, Musculoskeletal, and Neuromotor Fitness in Apparently Healthy Adults: Guidance for Prescribing Exercise : Medicine & Science in Sports & Exercise." LWW. Accessed October 29, 2015. http://journals.lww.com/acsm-msse/Fulltext/2011/07000/Quantity_and_Quality_of_Exercise_for_Developing.26.aspx.

4   "Leisure Time Physical Activity and Mortality: a Detailed Pooled Analysis of the Dose-response Relationship. - PubMed - NCBI." National Center for Biotechnology Information. Accessed October 29, 2015. http://www.ncbi.nlm.nih.gov/pubmed/25844730.

5   Adapted from Arem, H. et al, JAMA Intern Med, Accessed April 6, 2015. Doi: 10.1001/jamainternmed.2015.5033.

6   "Physical Activity Guidelines Health.gov." Accessed October 29, 2015. http://www.health.gov/paguidelines/.

7   "Associations Among Physical Activity, Diet Quality, and Weight Status in US Adults : Medicine & Science in Sports & Exercise." LWW. Accessed October 29, 2015. http://journals.lww.com/acsm-msse/Fulltext/2015/04000/Associations_among_Physical_Activity,_Diet.9.aspx.

8   Leong, Darryl P et al. "Prognostic value of grip strength: findings from the Prospective Urban Rural Epidemiology (PURE) study." The Lancet , Volume 386 , Issue 9990 , 266 – 273. Accessed October 29, 2015. http://www.thelancet.com/journals/lancet/article/PIIS0140-6736%2814%2962000-6/abstract.

9   "PLOS Medicine: Metabolic Signatures of Adiposity in Young Adults: Mendelian Randomization Analysis and Effects of Weight Change." Accessed October 29, 2015. http://journals.plos.org/plosmedicine/article?id=10.1371/journal.pmed.1001765.

10 National Heart, Lung, and Blood Institute (NHLBI) - NHLBI, NIH. Accessed October 29, 2015. http://www.nhlbi.nih.gov/health/educational/wecan/portion/documents/PD1.pdf.

11 "Portion Sizes - About Us - British Heart Foundation." We Fight for Every Heartbeat - British Heart Foundation. Accessed October 29, 2015. https://www.bhf.org.uk/about-us/our-policies/preventing-heart-disease/portion-sizes.aspx.

12 "Weight Loss Regulates Inflammation-related Genes in White Adipose Tissue of Obese Subjects." The FASEB Journal. Accessed October 29, 2015. http://www.fasebj. org/content/18/14/1657.full.

13 "PLOS Medicine: Metabolic Signatures of Adiposity in Young Adults: Mendelian Randomization Analysis and Effects of Weight Change." Accessed October 29, 2015. http://journals.plos.org/plosmedicine/article?id=10.1371/journal.pmed.1001765.

14 "Self-monitoring in Weight Loss: a Systematic Review of the Literature. - PubMed - NCBI." National Center for Biotechnology Information. Accessed October 29, 2015. http://www.ncbi.nlm.nih.gov/pubmed/21185970.

15 "BMR Calculator." BMI Calculator. Accessed October 29, 2015. http://www.bmi-calculator.net/bmr-calculator/.

16 "The Accuracy of Stated Energy Contents of Reduced-energy, Commercially Prepared Foods. - PubMed - NCBI." National Center for Biotechnology Information. Accessed October 29, 2015. http://www.ncbi.nlm.nih.gov/pubmed/20102837.

17 "A Human Thrifty Phenotype Associated With Less Weight Loss During Caloric Restriction." Diabetes. Accessed October 29, 2015. http://diabetes.diabetesjournals. org/content/early/2015/05/06/db14-1881.

18 Nature Publishing Group: Science Journals, Jobs, and Information. Accessed October 29, 2015. http://www.nature.com/ijo/journal/v32/n1/pdf/0803712a.pdf.

19 "Wake Up America : a National Sleep Alert : Report of the National Commission on Sleep Disorders Research (Microform, 1993) [WorldCat.org]." WorldCat.org: The World's Largest Library Catalog. Accessed October 29, 2015. http://www.worldcat. org/title/wake-up-america-a-national-sleep-alert-report-of-the-national-commission-on-sleep-disorders-research/oclc/34483350.

20 "2005 Sleep in America Poll: Summary of Findings." National Sleep Foundation. Accessed October 29, 2015. http://sleepfoundation.org/sites/default/files/2005_summary_of_findings.pdf.

21 "Extent and Health Consequences of Chronic Sleep Loss and Sleep Disorders - Sleep Disorders and Sleep Deprivation - NCBI Bookshelf." National Center for Biotechnology Information. Accessed October 29, 2015. http://www.ncbi.nlm.nih.gov/books/ NBK19961/.

22 "Insomnia with Short Sleep Duration and Mortality: The Penn State Cohort." PubMed Central (PMC). Accessed October 29, 2015. http://www.ncbi.nlm.nih.gov/ pmc/articles/PMC2938855/.

23 "Short Duration of Sleep Increases Risk of Colorectal Adenoma - Thompson - 2010 - Cancer." Wiley Online Library. Accessed October 29, 2015. http://onlinelibrary.wiley. com/doi/10.1002/cncr.25507/abstract.

24 "Association of Sleep Duration and Breast Cancer OncotypeDX Recurrence Score. - PubMed - NCBI." National Center for Biotechnology Information. Accessed October 29, 2015. http://www.ncbi.nlm.nih.gov/pubmed/22752291.

25 "Insufficient Sleep Undermines Dietary Efforts to Reduce Adiposity | Annals of Internal Medicine." Journal | Annals of Internal Medicine. Accessed October 29, 2015. http://annals.org/article.aspx?articleid=746184.

26 "The Impact of Sleep Deprivation on Food Desire in the Human Brain." PubMed Central (PMC). Accessed October 29, 2015. http://www.ncbi.nlm.nih.gov/pmc/articles/PMC3763921/.

27 "Sleep Loss Reduces Diurnal Rhythm Amplitude of Leptin in Healthy Men." Perelman School of Medicine at the University of Pennsylvania. Accessed October 29, 2015. http://depressiongenetics.med.upenn.edu/uep/user_documents/dfd13.pdf.

28 "Leptin Levels Are Dependent on Sleep Duration: Relationships with Sympathovagal Balance, Carbohydrate Regulation, Cortisol, and Thyrotropin. - PubMed - NCBI." National Center for Biotechnology Information. Accessed October 29, 2015. http://www.ncbi.nlm.nih.gov/pubmed/15531540.

29 "Sleep Duration and Body Mass Index in Twins: A Gene-Environment Interaction." PubMed Central (PMC). Accessed October 29, 2015. http://www.ncbi.nlm.nih.gov/pmc/articles/PMC3321418/.

30 "The Cumulative Cost of Additional Wakefulness: Dose-Response Effects on Neurobehavioral Functions and Sleep Physiology From Chronic Sleep Restriction and Total Sleep Deprivation." Perelman School of Medicine at the University of Pennsylvania. Accessed October 29, 2015. http://www.med.upenn.edu/uep/user_documents/VanDongen_etal_Sleep_26_2_2003.pdf.

31 "Cognitive Behavioral Therapy for Chronic Insomnia: A Systematic Review and Meta-analysisCognitive Behavioral Therapy for Chronic Insomnia | Annals of Internal Medicine." Journal | Annals of Internal Medicine. Accessed October 29, 2015. http://annals.org/article.aspx?articleid=2301405.

32 "Chronic Inflammation Induces Telomere Dysfunction and Accelerates Ageing in Mice : Nature Communications : Nature Publishing Group." Nature Publishing Group : Science Journals, Jobs, and Information. Accessed October 29, 2015. http://www.nature.com/ncomms/2014/140624/ncomms5172/full/ncomms5172.html.

33 "Caloric Restriction Reduces Age-related and All-cause Mortality in Rhesus Monkeys : Nature Communications : Nature Publishing Group." Nature Publishing Group : Science Journals, Jobs, and Information. Accessed October 29, 2015. http://www.nature.com/ncomms/2014/140401/ncomms4557/full/ncomms4557.html.

34   "Long-term Calorie Restriction is Highly Effective in Reducing the Risk for Athero-sclerosis in Humans." PubMed Central (PMC). Accessed October 29, 2015. http://www.ncbi.nlm.nih.gov/pmc/articles/PMC404101/.

35   "PLOS ONE: The Relationship Between Inflammatory Biomarkers and Telomere Length in an Occupational Prospective Cohort Study." Accessed October 29, 2015. http://journals.plos.org/plosone/article?id=10.1371/journal.pone.0087348.

36   "Inflammation and Cancer: Interweaving MicroRNA, Free Radical, Cytokine and P53 Pathways." PubMed Central (PMC). Accessed October 29, 2015. http://www.ncbi.nlm.nih.gov/pmc/articles/PMC2802675/.

37   Wiley Online Library. Accessed October 29, 2015. http://onlinelibrary.wiley.com/store/10.1080/15216540410001701642/asset/714309677_ftp.pdf;jsessionid=8D097FFDDE88BB0EC5C2FEF9599152C0.f04t01?v=1&t=iekm0do-q&s=7121a31b344ae50ec6bfcae4e7520abed5f2cc34.

38   "Physical Exercise and Cognitive Performance in the Elderly: Current Perspectives." PubMed Central (PMC). Accessed October 29, 2015. http://www.ncbi.nlm.nih.gov/pmc/articles/PMC3872007/.

39   "Cardiorespiratory Fitness and Cognitive Function in Middle Age: the CARDIA Study. - PubMed - NCBI." National Center for Biotechnology Information. Accessed October 29, 2015. http://www.ncbi.nlm.nih.gov/pubmed/24696506.

40   "Diet, Lifestyle, and the Risk of Type 2 Diabetes Mellitus in Women — NEJM." New England Journal of Medicine. Accessed October 29, 2015. http://www.nejm.org/doi/full/10.1056/NEJMoa010492.

41   "Effect of Potentially Modifiable Risk Factors Associated with Myocardial Infarction in 52 Countries (the INTERHEART Study): Case-control Study. - PubMed - NCBI." National Center for Biotechnology Information. Accessed October 29, 2015. http://www.ncbi.nlm.nih.gov/pubmed/15364185.

42   "Healthy Lifestyle Factors in the Primary Prevention of Coronary Heart Disease Among Men: Benefits Among Users and Nonusers of Lipid-lowering and Antihypertensive Medications - PubMed - NCBI." National Center for Biotechnology Information. Accessed October 29, 2015. http://www.ncbi.nlm.nih.gov/pubmed/16818808.

43   "Combined Effect of Low-risk Dietary and Lifestyle Behaviors in Primary Prevention of Myocardial Infarction in Women. - PubMed - NCBI." National Center for Biotechnology Information. Accessed October 29, 2015. http://www.ncbi.nlm.nih.gov/pubmed/17954808.

44   "Primary Prevention of Stroke by Healthy Lifestyle." Circulation. Accessed October 29, 2015. http://circ.ahajournals.org/content/118/9/947.full.

45 "Sufficient Sleep Duration Contributes to Lower Cardiovascular Disease Risk in Addition to Four Traditional Lifestyle Factors: the MORGEN Study. - PubMed - NCBI." National Center for Biotechnology Information. Accessed October 29, 2015. http://www.ncbi.nlm.nih.gov/pubmed/23823570.

46 American College of Cardiology Foundation | Journal of the American College of Cardiology | Journal. Accessed October 29, 2015. http://content.onlinejacc.org/article.aspx?articleid=1909605.

47 "Social Networks, Host Resistance, and Mortality: A Nine-year Follow-up Study of Alameda County Residents." Oxford Journals | Medicine & Health | American Jnl of Epidemiology. Accessed October 29, 2015. http://aje.oxfordjournals.org/content/109/2/186.short.

48 "JAMA Network | JAMA Psychiatry | Emotional Vitality and Incident Coronary Heart Disease: Benefits of Healthy Psychological Functioning." JAMA Network | JAMA Psychiatry | Home. Accessed October 29, 2015. http://archpsyc.jamanetwork.com/article.aspx?articleid=482515.

49 "Triumphs of Experience — George E. Vaillant | Harvard University Press." Home | Harvard University Press. Accessed October 29, 2015. http://www.hup.harvard.edu/catalog.php?isbn=9780674059825.

50 "Social Networks, Host Resistance, and Mortality: A Nine-year Follow-up Study of Alameda County Residents." Oxford Journals | Medicine & Health | American Jnl of Epidemiology. Accessed October 29, 2015. http://aje.oxfordjournals.org/content/109/2/186.short.

51 "PLOS Medicine: Social Relationships and Mortality Risk: A Meta-analytic Review." Accessed October 29, 2015. http://journals.plos.org/plosmedicine/article?id=10.1371/journal.pmed.1000316.

52 "The Pittsburgh Common Cold Studies: Psychosocial predictors of susceptibility to respiratory infectious illness." Research Showcase @ CMU. Accessed October 29, 2015. http://repository.cmu.edu/cgi/viewcontent.cgi?article=1273&context=psychology.

53 "Stress, Personal Relationships, and Immune Function: Health Implications." Psychoneuroimmunology Research Program. Accessed October 29, 2015. http://pni.osumc.edu/KG%20Publications%20(pdf)/130.pdf.

54 "JAMA Network | JAMA Psychiatry | Emotional Vitality and Incident Coronary Heart Disease: Benefits of Healthy Psychological Functioning." JAMA Network | JAMA Psychiatry | Home. Accessed October 29, 2015. http://archpsyc.jamanetwork.com/article.aspx?articleid=482515.

55 "PLOS ONE: Giving Leads to Happiness in Young Children." Accessed October 29, 2015. http://journals.plos.org/plosone/article?id=10.1371/journal.pone.0039211.

56   "The Paradox of Generosity: Giving We Receive, Grasping We Lose: Christian Smith, Hilary Davidson: 9780199394906: Amazon.com: Books." Amazon.com: Online Shopping for Electronics, Apparel, Computers, Books, DVDs & More. Accessed October 29, 2015. http://www.amazon.com/Paradox-Generosity-Giving-Receive-Grasping/dp/0199394903/ref=sr_1_1?ie=UTF8&qid=1410659309&sr=8-1&keywords=the+paradox+of+generosity.

57   "JAMA Network | JAMA Pediatrics | Effect of Volunteering on Risk Factors for Cardiovascular Disease in Adolescents: A Randomized Controlled Trial." JAMA Network | JAMA Pediatrics | Home. Accessed October 29, 2015. http://archpedi.jama-network.com/article.aspx?articleid=1655500&resultClick=3.

58   "Prosocial Foundations of Children's Academic Achievement." University of Kentucky. Accessed October 29, 2015. http://www.uky.edu/~eushe2/BanduraPubs/Bandura2000PS.pdf.

59   "The Science of Generosity." Psychology Today. Accessed October 29, 2015. https://www.psychologytoday.com/blog/the-moral-molecule/200911/the-science-generosity.

60   "Happiness Runs in a Circular Motion: Evidence for a Positive Feedback Loop Between Prosocial Spending and Happiness - Article." Harvard Business School. Accessed October 29, 2015. http://www.hbs.edu/faculty/Pages/item.aspx?num=42426.

61   "Blue Zones – Dan Buettner." Blue Zones. Accessed October 29, 2015. https://www.bluezones.com/speaking/dan-buettner/.

62   "Abstract 52: Purpose in Life and Its Relationship to All-Cause Mortality and Cardiovascular Events: A Meta-Analysis." Circulation. Accessed October 29, 2015. http://circ.ahajournals.org/content/131/Suppl_1/A52.abstract?sid=4f4f8747-5eab-4ade-9115-3e97afc90c13.

63   "Purpose in Life As a Predictor of Mortality Across Adulthood." Psychological Science. Accessed October 29, 2015. http://pss.sagepub.com/content/25/7/1482.

64   Steptoe, Andrew et al. "Subjective wellbeing, health, and ageing." The Lancet, Volume 385, Issue 9968, 640 – 648. Accessed October 29, 2015. http://www.thelancet.com/journals/lancet/article/PIIS0140-6736(13)61489-0/abstract.

65   "Purpose in Life Is Associated With Mortality Among Community-Dwelling Older Persons." PubMed Central (PMC). Accessed October 29, 2015. http://www.ncbi.nlm.nih.gov/pmc/articles/PMC2740716/.

66   "Purpose in Life and Use of Preventive Health Care Services." Proceedings of the National Academy of Sciences. Accessed October 29, 2015. http://www.pnas.org/content/111/46/16331.abstract.

67   "Abstract 52: Purpose in Life and Its Relationship to All-Cause Mortality and Cardio-vascular Events: A Meta-Analysis." Circulation. Accessed October 29, 2015. http://circ.ahajournals.org/content/131/Suppl_1/A52.abstract?sid=4f4f8747-5eab-4ade-9115-3e97afc90c13.

68   "Purpose in Life and Cerebral Infarcts in Community-Dwelling Older People." Stroke. Accessed October 29, 2015. http://stroke.ahajournals.org/content/46/4/1071.abstract.

69   "Overview and Findings from the Rush Memory and Aging Project." PubMed Central (PMC). Accessed October 29, 2015. http://www.ncbi.nlm.nih.gov/pmc/articles/PMC3439198/.

70   "Effect of a Purpose in Life on Risk of Incident Alzheimer Disease and Mild Cognitive Impairment in Community-Dwelling Older Persons." PubMed Central (PMC). Accessed October 29, 2015. http://www.ncbi.nlm.nih.gov/pmc/articles/PMC2897172/.

71   "JAMA Network | JAMA Psychiatry | Effect of Purpose in Life on the Relation Between Alzheimer Disease Pathologic Changes on Cognitive Function in Advanced Age." JAMA Network | JAMA Psychiatry | Home. Accessed October 29, 2015. http://archpsyc.jamanetwork.com/article.aspx?articleid=1151486.

72   "Understanding the Connection Between Spiritual Well-being and Physical Health: an Examination of Ambulatory Blood Pressure, Inflammation, Blood Lipids and Fasting Glucose - Springer." Home - Springer. Accessed October 29, 2015. http://link.springer.com/article/10.1007/s10865-011-9343-7#page-1.

73   "Positive Affect, Psychological Well-being, and Good Sleep. - PubMed - NCBI." National Center for Biotechnology Information. Accessed October 29, 2015. http://www.ncbi.nlm.nih.gov/pubmed/18374740.

74   "Sustained Striatal Activity Predicts Eudaimonic Well-being and Cortisol Output. - PubMed - NCBI." National Center for Biotechnology Information. Accessed October 29, 2015. http://www.ncbi.nlm.nih.gov/pubmed/24058063.

75   "A Functional Genomic Perspective on Human Well-being." Proceedings of the National Academy of Sciences. Accessed October 29, 2015. http://www.pnas.org/content/110/33/13684.abstract.

76   "Compound Facial Expressions of Emotion." Proceedings of the National Academy of Sciences. Accessed October 29, 2015. http://www.pnas.org/content/111/15/E1454.

77   Charles Darwin: The Expression of the Emotions in Man and Animals. New York: D. Appleton and Company (1872): 347-366.

78   "Awe, the Small Self, and Prosocial Behavior." Accessed October 29, 2015. http://www.apa.org/pubs/journals/releases/psp-pspi0000018.pdf.

79   Peterson, C.; Maier, S. F.; Seligman, M. E. P. (1995). Learned Helplessness: A Theory for the Age of Personal Control. New York: Oxford University Press.

80   Seligman, Martin. Learned Optimism. New York, NY: Pocket Books. 1998

CPSIA information can be obtained
at www.ICGtesting.com
Printed in the USA
LVOW05*0708201215

467127LV00009B/12/P